ASSESSING INITIATIVES TO INCREASE ORGAN DONATIONS

HEARING

BEFORE THE

SUBCOMMITTEE ON
OVERSIGHT AND INVESTIGATIONS

OF THE

COMMITTEE ON ENERGY AND COMMERCE
HOUSE OF REPRESENTATIVES

ONE HUNDRED EIGHTH CONGRESS

FIRST SESSION

JUNE 3, 2003

Serial No. 108–36

Printed for the use of the Committee on Energy and Commerce

Available via the World Wide Web: http://www.access.gpo.gov/congress/house

U.S. GOVERNMENT PRINTING OFFICE

87–490PDF   WASHINGTON : 2003

For sale by the Superintendent of Documents, U.S. Government Printing Office
Internet: bookstore.gpo.gov   Phone: toll free (866) 512–1800; DC area (202) 512–1800
Fax: (202) 512–2250   Mail: Stop SSOP, Washington, DC 20402–0001

COMMITTEE ON ENERGY AND COMMERCE

W.J. "BILLY" TAUZIN, Louisiana, *Chairman*

MICHAEL BILIRAKIS, Florida
JOE BARTON, Texas
FRED UPTON, Michigan
CLIFF STEARNS, Florida
PAUL E. GILLMOR, Ohio
JAMES C. GREENWOOD, Pennsylvania
CHRISTOPHER COX, California
NATHAN DEAL, Georgia
RICHARD BURR, North Carolina
  Vice Chairman
ED WHITFIELD, Kentucky
CHARLIE NORWOOD, Georgia
BARBARA CUBIN, Wyoming
JOHN SHIMKUS, Illinois
HEATHER WILSON, New Mexico
JOHN B. SHADEGG, Arizona
CHARLES W. "CHIP" PICKERING,
  Mississippi
VITO FOSSELLA, New York
ROY BLUNT, Missouri
STEVE BUYER, Indiana
GEORGE RADANOVICH, California
CHARLES F. BASS, New Hampshire
JOSEPH R. PITTS, Pennsylvania
MARY BONO, California
GREG WALDEN, Oregon
LEE TERRY, Nebraska
ERNIE FLETCHER, Kentucky
MIKE FERGUSON, New Jersey
MIKE ROGERS, Michigan
DARRELL E. ISSA, California
C.L. "BUTCH" OTTER, Idaho

JOHN D. DINGELL, Michigan
  Ranking Member
HENRY A. WAXMAN, California
EDWARD J. MARKEY, Massachusetts
RALPH M. HALL, Texas
RICK BOUCHER, Virginia
EDOLPHUS TOWNS, New York
FRANK PALLONE, Jr., New Jersey
SHERROD BROWN, Ohio
BART GORDON, Tennessee
PETER DEUTSCH, Florida
BOBBY L. RUSH, Illinois
ANNA G. ESHOO, California
BART STUPAK, Michigan
ELIOT L. ENGEL, New York
ALBERT R. WYNN, Maryland
GENE GREEN, Texas
KAREN McCARTHY, Missouri
TED STRICKLAND, Ohio
DIANA DeGETTE, Colorado
LOIS CAPPS, California
MICHAEL F. DOYLE, Pennsylvania
CHRISTOPHER JOHN, Louisiana
TOM ALLEN, Maine
JIM DAVIS, Florida
JAN SCHAKOWSKY, Illinois
HILDA L. SOLIS, California

DAN R. BROUILLETTE, *Staff Director*
JAMES D. BARNETTE, *General Counsel*
REID P.F. STUNTZ, *Minority Staff Director and Chief Counsel*

———

SUBCOMMITTEE ON OVERSIGHT AND INVESTIGATIONS

JAMES C. GREENWOOD, Pennsylvania, *Chairman*

MICHAEL BILIRAKIS, Florida
CLIFF STEARNS, Florida
RICHARD BURR, North Carolina
CHARLES F. BASS, New Hampshire
GREG WALDEN, Oregon
  Vice Chairman
MIKE FERGUSON, New Jersey
MIKE ROGERS, Michigan
W.J. "BILLY" TAUZIN, Louisiana
  (Ex Officio)

PETER DEUTSCH, Florida
  Ranking Member
DIANA DeGETTE, Colorado
JIM DAVIS, Florida
JAN SCHAKOWSKY, Illinois
HENRY A. WAXMAN, California
BOBBY L. RUSH, Illinois
JOHN D. DINGELL, Michigan,
  (Ex Officio)

(II)

CONTENTS

Page

ASSESSING INITIATIVES TO INCREASE ORGAN DONATIONS

TUESDAY, JUNE 3, 2003

HOUSE OF REPRESENTATIVES,
COMMITTEE ON ENERGY AND COMMERCE,
SUBCOMMITTEE ON OVERSIGHT AND INVESTIGATIONS,
Washington, DC.

The subcommittee met, pursuant to notice, at 10 a.m., in room 2322, Rayburn House Office Building, Hon. James C. Greenwood (chairman) presiding.

Members present: Representatives Greenwood, Bass, Walden, Ferguson, Tauzin (ex officio), Deutsch, and DeGette.

Staff present: Casey Hemard, majority counsel; Jill Latham, legislative clerk; David Nelson, minority counsel; and Nicole Kenner, Legislative analyst.

Mr. GREENWOOD. The subcommittee will come to order and the Chair recognizes himself for an opening statement.

Before then, without objection, the subcommittee will proceed pursuant to committee rule 4(c). So ordered. The Chair recognizes himself for an opening statement.

Good morning and welcome, everyone. It has been nearly 50 years since the first successful kidney transplant was performed in the United States. Since that first operation, the transplant community has developed into a national network of organ procurement organizations and 257 transplant centers where lifesaving operations are performed on a daily basis. Last year alone, 24,581 transplant operations were performed. Yet, despite this remarkable achievement, tens of thousands of people are waiting at any given moment for their chance at a lifesaving organ transplant. In 2002 alone, approximately 40,000 names were added to the waiting list. Just an hour ago the number of people waiting for organs was 81,752. Sadly, many of these people will run out of time. Last year, 6,187 people died while on the waiting list because there were simply not enough organs to meet demand.

What is particularly frustrating about these numbers, these missed chances to save a life, is that we know more organs could be made available. The Department of Health and Human Services recently reviewed national data from the Organ Procurement and Transplantation Network Data base and found that only 40 percent of individuals who died and had organs eligible for donation actually became donors.

When you consider that as many as eight lives can be saved from the gifts of one donor and that there are more than 81,000 people needing a lifesaving organ, 40 percent is just not good enough.

(1)

These numbers demonstrate that initiatives being undertaken in this country to educate people on the merits of organ donation are failing to meet the ever-growing demand for organs. What is the solution to this dilemma?

This morning we will hear from members of the organ donation community who will help us find some potential answers. We will hear about new measures and initiatives that hold some promise for increasing donation rates. We will learn more about what is being done with the organ transplant community at the local State and national levels.

First we will hear those most affected by the current organ donation process. On the first panel, we will meet Reginald Augustus, a 27-year-old man who has been waiting for a kidney transplant for the past 2 years. Reginald will tell us about the complications he faces on a daily basis as he juggles everyday life with the limitation of dialysis.

We will meet Chris and Cheryl Koller of Cary, North Carolina. The Kollers are parents of 10-year-old Caitlyn Koller—good morning, Caitlyn—who received a lifesaving heart transplant when she was just 8 years old, and she has a birthday coming up in January.

The choice to give up your loved one's organs is a heroic one. This morning we will also hear from Susan Kantrowitz, one such hero, to help us understand the struggles she went through in making the decision to donate the organs of her late husband William.

Rounding out our first panel will be Joseph Roth from the Organ Procurement Organizations. Organ procurement organizations, known as OPOs, are responsible for coordinating the organ transplant process at the community level. Mr. Roth will discuss how OPOs facilitate the process of getting donor organs to those in need.

It is encouraging to see the Bush Administration has been addressing this issue. Health and Human Services Secretary Tommy Thompson has made public awareness about organ donation a priority. In late 2002, Secretary Thompson's Advisory Committee on Organ Transplantation made 18 recommendations relating to organ donation and transplant issues.

And on the hearing's second panel this morning, Michelle Snyder, director of HHS's Office of Special Programs will discuss those recommendations and how they will affect the organ donor process. She will address the best practices initiatives that HHS has undertaken in the past year to identify organ donation practices at the most effective hospitals and transfer them to underperforming institutions to help increase the number of donors nationwide.

Ms. Snyder will be joined by Doctor Bob Metzger, President-elect of the United Network for Organ Sharing, or UNOS, who can explain to us how UNOS facilitates the organ-matching and procurement process throughout the country. UNOS is the organization that holds the contract for the Organ Procurement and Transplantation Network.

Our third panel will allow us to expand our inquiry to new research and other approaches that may help increase the availability of lifesaving organs for those in need. We will hear from Tim Olsen, the Community Development Coordinator at the Wisconsin Donor Network, where his organ procurement organization has had one of the largest increases in donations in the country last year.

Dr. Jay Vacanti, Director of Pediatric Transplantation at Massachusetts General Hospital, will describe some of the advances in research that have been made to provide other options to individuals in need of organs.

And Doctor Abraham Shaked, President of the American Society of Transplant Surgeons, will discuss solutions that the society has explored.

Another important issue this hearing will explore today is the current Federal prohibition on payments to donors for their organs. The National Organ Transplant Act prohibits the sale or purchase of human organs. However, frustrated by the alarming shortage of donor organs, many in the medical community have begun to question whether it might be possible to provide some sort of ethically acceptable financial incentive to the beneficiaries of a decedent that may motivate an individual to formally express his intentions about donation prior to his or her death.

Given that so many people die each year waiting for an organ transplant, I believe all options should be put on the table as we discuss ways to increase organ donations. In this regard, we will receive testimony from Rich DeVos, a heart transplant recipient, who will discuss how providing insurance benefits or a tax credit to cadaveric donors may both increase donations and save insurers and Medicare money.

And Dr. Robert Sade will be here on behalf of the American Medical Association to discuss a policy the Association adopted last summer to encourage study of the use of financial incentives to increase cadaveric organ donation.

However, the National Kidney Foundation has voiced its opposition to any sort of financial incentives for donation, and Doctor Francis Delmonico will be here to explain that position as well.

Clearly we have many complicated and sensitive issues to examine this morning, and let me thank all the witnesses for attending this important hearing. And I turn now to recognize the ranking member for his opening statement.

Mr. DEUTSCH. I yield my time.

Mr. GREENWOOD. The ranking member yields his time to the gentlelady from Colorado, who is recognized for 5 minutes.

Ms. DEGETTE. Thank you very much, Mr. Chairman. I am very pleased that we are having this hearing today to assess various initiatives that the Federal Government and its agencies have undertaken to increase organ donation. We all know that organ donation save lives. Every day, about 63 people receive an organ transplant; but unfortunately another 16 people who are on the waiting list die because not enough organs are available.

So the question of what role the government should play in increasing the organ donations is an important one. Overall the national outlook for organ donations is not particularly rosy. The number of people awaiting organ transplants is up and the amount of time patients must wait for an organ transplant is also increasing.

I am very interested in the state of organ donations and transplants because I am the co-chair of the House Caucus on Diabetes and I understand the life-giving nature of kidney transplants for patients with renal failure. I am also interested in organ donation because my bill in the 106th Congress, which one of our witnesses will be particularly interested in today, the Pediatric Organ Transplantation Act, was fully incorporated into law as part of H.R. 4365, the Children's Health Act of 2000. What the legislation did was require the Organ Transplantation Network to adopt criteria, policies, and procedures to address the unique health care needs of children. In addition, the legislation required a study of the unique health care needs of children, including growth and developmental issues and immunosuppressant drug coverage and organ transplantation. The study was intended to give a more complete picture of the full-range picture of problems in pediatric organ transplantation.

I am going to be very interested during the course of the testimony today to hear what kind of progress has been made in advancing the cause of pediatric organ transplantation and making sure that kids who are on waiting lists get pediatric organs.

I would like to make one final note. It has been against the public policy of this country to pay people for organ donations for many, many years, and the reason is because legislative bodies have felt that it was repugnant to give financial incentives to folks to donate their own organs, and the feeling is that it would unduly put pressure on low-income individuals to do that.

I see no need to move away from that public policy. In fact, in light of recent tax cut policies and other financial policies of this administration, it seems to me we are giving less and less relief to low-income individuals and more and more tax relief to high-income individuals. I don't see why we would even do a study at this point to give financial incentives for lower-income people to have to sell their organs, and I am very much opposed to even doing a study on that idea. I think it would be discriminatory toward low-income people.

When you couple that with studies that we have seen that indicate that other kinds of incentives, like education programs through the States where we could put Federal resources to work, I don't see any reason to give financial incentives to individuals for organ donation. I think it is always interesting to discuss issues, but I would be appalled by any legislative efforts to change our longstanding policy. And I think, frankly, most experts, certainly in organ transplantation, would also be opposed to this issue. I just put that out.

I am eager to hear the testimony and I want to thank all of our witnesses for coming. I know that it is particularly difficult for 10-year-olds to come and testify before Congress, but the kind of testimony that you can give us is really going to help us in our deliberations. So thank you so much, and I yield back.

Mr. GREENWOOD. Thank the gentlelady. Actually, I think Caitlyn looks more relaxed than anyone else.

The Chair recognizes the gentleman, Mr. Walden, for an opening statement.

Mr. WALDEN. Thank you, Mr. Chairman, and thank you for convening this hearing.

The fact that advances in medicine and science have brought us to a point where organs from one individual can be transplanted into another successfully is extraordinary and remarkable. It is also very complicated and involved, not only in the short term but the long term.

In my home State of Oregon, there are 376 Oregonians who are waiting organ transplants. These aren't just numbers, they are sons and daughters and wives and husbands and mothers and fathers, and I applaud those who have signed up to be organ donors.

I apologize if I am a little emotional. Nine years ago and 5 months, we lost our second son who was awaiting an organ donation. He came premature, and we were never able to see through the surgery, which we planned to have at Loma Linda, for a heart transplant. He suffered from Hypoplastic Left Heart Syndrome.

I am very dedicated to doing whatever we can to encourage and facilitate the donations of organs. I know what it means to families to be a recipient. I know how difficult, or at least I can only imagine how difficult it is for those who have loved ones who have to donate or are allowed to donate. I prefer to think of it as allowing to donate so another can live or see.

And I don't want to get into arguments of class warfare. I want to get into figuring out how to improve the system so no parent has to watch and wait until their loved one dies while we argue and debate. Obviously, we have to do it in a proper and appropriate way. We don't want to create an ugly incentive to do bad things. We want to do good things. And so I commend the medical community for the advancements that have taken place. I encourage additional scientific review. And certainly what we all, or a lot of us, do to sign up to be organ donors on our driver's license I think is really helpful.

So, Mr. Chairman, I appreciate this hearing and I look forward to working with you on these efforts.

Mr. GREENWOOD. I thank the gentleman for his statement and his candor.

The gentleman from New Jersey is recognized.

Mr. FERGUSON. Thank you, Mr. Chairman. I, too, am a great supporter of organ donation. In fact, I was on my way walking over to this hearing. I just got a replacement license a few days ago and I had not turned it over, signed the back of it, and checked off my organ donor box. So if nothing else, this hearing did some good to remind one person to renew their commitment to organ donation.

It is imperative, obviously, that we increase organ donation in our country. Unfortunately, our organ donation system is not providing enough donor organs to satisfy the life-sustaining demand we have in our country. There are more than 81,000 people in the U.S. Waiting to receive an organ transplant. For those people waiting for a transplant, fewer than a third of them will receive a transplant this year. Every 13 minutes another name is added to the transplant waiting list, with approximately 40,000 names that were added to the waiting list last year in 2002 alone. Tragically, a staggering average of 16 people a day are lost because they can't be matched with an organ donor in time, adding up to more than 6,000 people who were lost last year waiting for a transplant.

Our doctors and those who administer the Organ Donor Networks already do an incredible job, saving as many lives as they can under the current circumstances. However, we have to look deeper into the matter and we have to work hard to make sure the system is more efficient to increase the number of donations that are made available. Our goal should be that these people who are seeking donor organs and those donating organs achieve parity as soon as possible.

Today we will consider several initiatives and we will hear from our witnesses and others who have sought to improve organ donation and transmission. And I look forward to hearing about some of the successes, too, of these programs and any suggestions that our panelists may have to make the environment better for organ donation.

Thank you, Mr. Chairman. I thank all of our panelists today and I look forward to the hearing.

Mr. GREENWOOD. The Chair thanks the gentleman.

[Additional statement submitted for the record follows:]

PREPARED STATEMENT OF HON. BOBBY L. RUSH, A REPRESENTATIVE IN CONGRESS FROM THE STATE OF ILLINOIS

Mr. Chairman: I applaud the Subcommittee for holding this important hearing on the status of organ donations in the United States. With more than 81,000 critically ill people in the United States currently waiting to receive a transplant this year, this hearing is both timely and appropriate.

In 1984, Congress enacted the National Organ Transplant Act which created the Organ Procurement and Transplantation Network (OPTN), designed to increase the supply of viable organs available for transplant. Under the provisions of the National Organ Transplant Act (NOTA), the U.S. Department of Health and Human Services has the responsibility for establishing and administering a national organ allocation program, through its prime contractor, UNOS.

In 2000, HHS established an Advisory Committee on Organ Transplantation to advise the Secretary on all issues related to organ donation and in November of last year, the Committee made a number of recommendations—18—to the Secretary relating to the treatment of both living and deceased organ donors.

Several of the recommendations promulgated by the Advisory Committee are issues which my good friend and colleague, Ray LaHood, and I attempted to address in legislation which we sponsored in the 106th Congress. As introduced, H.R. 3885 was designed to increase organ donation by establishing a grant program to assist organ procurement organizations (OPO) and other non-profit organizations in developing and expanding programs aimed at increasing organ donation rates; creating a Congressional Donor Medal to be awarded to living organ donors or to organ donor families; establishing a system of accountability and placing the responsibility for increasing organ donation with the Department of Health and Human Services (HHS must report its progress to Congress); and establishing a system of support for state programs to increase organ donation. Although Congress did not pass H.R. 3885, the dialogue which was initiated around that bill resulted in several improvements to the donation and allocation system.

Mr. Chairman, I am pleased that this Subcommittee will address some of these issues today.

Mr. GREENWOOD. And now we turn to our witnesses. And they are: Mr. Reginald Augustus from Gaithersburg, Maryland; Ms. Susan Kantrowitz—am I pronouncing that correctly—from Alexandria, Virginia; Ms. Cheryl Koller and her daughter Caitlyn from Cary, North Carolina; and Mr. Joseph Roth, President-elect of the Association of Organ Procurement Organizations in McLean, Virginia.

Thank you for being with us this morning. I think you have been informed that this is an investigative hearing. And when we hold investigative hearings it is our custom to take testimony under oath, and I ask if you object to giving your testimony under oath. And then I need to tell you are permitted, pursuant to our rules, to be represented by counsel.

Do any of you wish to be represented by counsel? Didn't think so. In that case, if you would stand and raise your right hands, I will give you the oath.

[Witnesses sworn.]

Mr. GREENWOOD. You may be seated, and are under oath, and we will begin with Mr. Augustus. And you are recognized for your opening statement.

TESTIMONY OF REGINALD AUGUSTUS; SUSAN KANTROWITZ; CHERYL KOLLER, PARENT OF CAITLYN, SUCCESSFUL TRANSPLANT RECIPIENT; JOSEPH ROTH, PRESIDENT-ELECT, ASSOCIATION OF ORGAN PROCUREMENT ORGANIZATIONS

Mr. AUGUSTUS. Good morning. My name is Reginald Augustus, and I'm here to tell you about my life and how it has been, dealing with kidney failure while waiting for a kidney transplant. In May 1999, during a routine physical, my doctor told me that my kidneys were not functioning properly. On that day, my life changed forever. As time went on, I began not to feel well. My blood pressure began to elevate and I felt shortness of breath and I would feel nauseous often. By the time I went back to the doctor in March 2001, I needed to be put on emergency dialysis, given two blood transfusions, and had to spend 5 days in the hospital.

Since March 2001, I have been on kidney dialysis. I had to change a lot of things such as my diet. I now have to watch certain foods and fluids that are high in potassium, which could cause a heart attack, high-phosphorus foods which eventually could thin my bones and make them brittle, and also have to watch my fluid intake which could eventually get into my lungs. My body no longer gets rid of these fluids like a normal person would. And I have to watch those types of things.

I have to go about three times a week to kidney dialysis, where I get stuck with two large needles into my arm where surgery was performed, called a fitula, and that is where an artery and a vein are connected to make the vein large enough to handle the blood being pumped through a filter, which is called dialyzer, and it cleans my blood and takes out excess fluids. Not only is this process inconvenient, lasting about 4 hours per treatment, but it also leaves me feeling worn out afterwards.

Many dialysis patients such as myself cramp badly from fluids taken off, and we have to deal with our blood pressure dropping, stripping out of our bodies not only toxins but minerals and chemicals and vitamins that our body needs. The process of dialysis affects one's body in a negative way. Long periods of time on dialysis will shorten a person's life.

Other than dialysis, going about my daily activities, I don't feel the same as I used to. I get tired faster as the toxins in my body don't have anywhere to go. They buildup and kill red blood cells.

At the dialysis center, I get epogen medication to help produce red blood cells, which my kidneys once did for me. I also get a medication called Zemplar to help control my phosphorus and potassium levels and my parathyroid.

I have met many people at the dialysis center, some of whom have been on dialysis for a short time, some for a very long time. The ones who have been on for several years look different than the newer ones. Years of dialysis and kidney failure have darkened their skin and made them look weak and sickly. My uncle spent 20-plus years on dialysis before dying in his early forties, and I watched his body deteriorate and his bones become brittle, and was basically a hunched-over shell of a man at the end.

For many, work is not an option. Many work part time or not at all, because they are on dialysis. Every day, more and more people go on dialysis and the need is even greater for organ donation. Currently I believe the national average wait is somewhere over $3\frac{1}{2}$ years, and that is even longer for African Americans. I have been on the waiting list for 2 years, but I know many have been waiting twice as long as I have. The need again for organs is great and we need to increase the availability.

Thank you for your time. And I just want to put one more note on that. Kidney dialysis is available to me. Unfortunately, for some people who are waiting for organ donations and on lists, they need to get it sooner. I have something that can sustain me until the time is right, but people who are waiting for heart, lung, liver, the need is very great for them.

[The prepared statement of Reginald Augustus follows:]

PREPARED STATEMENT OF REGINALD AUGUSTUS

Hello, my name is Reginald Augustus and I am here today to tell you about how my life been dealing with kidney failure while waiting for a kidney transplant. In May of 1999, during a routine physical, my doctor told me my kidney's were not functioning properly. On that day my life changed forever. As time went on I began to not feel well. My blood pressure began to elevate, I felt shortness of breath, and I would feel nauseous often. By the time I went back to the doctor in March of 2001, I needed to be put on emergency dialysis, given 2 blood transfusions, and I had to spend 5 days in the hospital. Since March of 2001, I've been on kidney dialysis. I had to change a lot of things such as my diet. I now have to watch certain foods and fluids that are high in potassium which could cause a heart attack, high phosphorous foods which could eventually thin my bones and make them brittle. I also have to watch my fluid intake, since my body no longer gets ridof this fluid which can cause problems by getting into my lungs which has happened and around my heart which can lead to other problems. I also have to go 3 times a week for kidney dialysis where I get stuck with 2 large needles into my arm where a surgery was performed called a fistula where an artery and a vein are connected to make the vein large enough to handle your blood being sucked out and pumped through a filter (dialyzer) that cleans my blood and takes out excess fluid. Not only is this process inconvenient, lasting about 4 hours per treatment, but it leaves me feeling worn out afterwards. Many dialysis patients such as myself, cramp badly from the fluids being taken off. We also have to deal with our blood pressure dropping and the stripping out of our bodies not just toxins, but minerals and vitamins are bodies need. The process of dialysis effects ones body in a negative way. Long periods of time on dialysis will shorten a persons life. Other than dialysis, going about my day to day activities, I don't feel the same as I use to. I get tired faster as the toxins in my body don't have anywhere to go. They build up and kill red blood cells. At the dialysis center, I get epogen medication to help produce red red blood cells which my kidney's once did for me. I also get a medication called Zemplar, to help control my phosphorous and calcium levels and my parathyroid. I've met many people at the dialysis center. Some who have been on dialysis a short time and some a very long time. The ones who have been on for several years look different than the newer ones. Years of dialysis and kidney failure have darkened there skin and made them weak and sickly looking. My uncle spent 20 plus years on dialysis before dying in his early 40's. I watched his body deteriorate, his bones become brittle, and was basically a hunched over shell of a man at the end. For many, work is not an option. Many work part time or not at all because of dialysis. Everyday more and more people go on dialysis and the need is greater than ever for organ donation. Currently, I believe the national average wait is over 3½ years and it's even longer for African-Americans. I've been on the waiting list for 2 years but many I know have been waiting more than twice as long as me. The need for organs is great and we need to increase there availability. Thank you for your time.

Mr. GREENWOOD. We thank you for your testimony and your courage and candor as well.

Ms. Kantrowitz

TESTIMONY OF SUSAN KANTROWITZ

Ms. KANTROWITZ. Good morning. My name is Susan Kantrowitz. I am here speaking on behalf of myself. My husband Bill was a deceased donor, and I am here to tell you my story. It is indeed my pleasure.

For us it was an ordinary Friday night. My mother came for Friday night. My mother came to dinner. My 4-year-old was bouncing off the walls and my 1-year-old was trying to do a little furniture surfing as he was learning how to walk. And we had dinner, and my husband changed and he went back to work. He was the Deputy Chief Counsel for the Bureau of Engraving and Printing and needed to take a deposition from someone on the night shift.

We had an ordinary evening. I went to bed. I got up around midnight with the baby. Got him back to bed. Bill had come in and I went down to see him. He normally put his notes in the computer in the basement before he retired in the evening. When I went down there, I found Bill on the floor. It was obvious he had laid down and put a toy beneath his head. I thought he was snoring and I hesitated for 1 minute to think, well, maybe I will let him sleep there; but, you know, the basement is pretty cold so I decided I would go down and wake him up. When I went over, it was obvious there was a problem. I couldn't wake him up, and I called 911 immediately.

We live about a block, if that, from Mount Vernon Hospital. So when the paramedics came, they gave me a choice of walking over or going with them. I called the neighbor to stay with the kids and I went on my way. As I was walking out of the house, a paramedic came to me and said, "There is something going on," and he pointed to his head, indicating that Bill had a problem somewhere in his mind or his brain.

As I was walking toward the hospital, I met my neighbor. He gave me a cell phone and stayed with me so I wouldn't be alone. So I stayed for awhile; I am sure it was several hours by the time the nurse came in. She told me that a CT scan had revealed that Bill had had a stroke, that there was blood in his brain. It was pretty massive. They called the neurosurgeon. After the neurosurgeon took a look at Bill and examined him, he called me into his room and showed me the CT scan, which to me was like looking at Greek, and we talked a little bit. He tried to show me Bill had no responses, but I didn't really understand that. I was in the midst of a tragedy. We went through his particular case. The neurosurgeon basically said that he wouldn't operate, that there was no hope, that he didn't think he could save Bill's life, and if he could save Bill's life, that there would be no quality of life.

We started the discussion at that point about organ donation. That discussion lasted at least a full day. Just at the moment that they talked to me about organ donation, I had a flashback. Bill and I—and this was way before we had children—had the TV on, and on came an old episode of ER. And in this episode there was a teenage girl who had cystic fibrosis and needed a lung transplant to live, and in the next room there was a fireman who had been burned severely and was going to die. And as Hollywood would have it, it was the perfect match for this teenage girl, but he wasn't dead yet. And there was an incredible discussion in this episode about whether they could hasten the death of the firefighter in order to give the girl the transplant.

I remember this like it was yesterday. I remember it because the next morning we actually talked about this episode on our way to work, and Bill said to me, I can't believe how irresponsible that is, to actually imply that a doctor would take the life of another so that he could transplant an organ into a person who is going to live.

We talked about it for quite awhile on our way to work. And we agreed that if it ever came to pass, we would gladly give each other's organs. So even though I was remembering this conversation and even though that I knew that Bill consented to the organ transplant, I hesitated. My husband was lying in front of me. He was breathing. His heart was beating. His kidneys were working. He was sweating. It was warm on an August evening. And I really felt like I was sending him to his death, that I was somehow turning my back on him.

Luckily I have a brother-in-law who is a doctor. He looked at other things. He reiterated, Bill's not coming back, he's gone. The coordinator for the Washington Regional Transplant Organization was wonderful. He talked me through a million questions: What were you going to take—how are you going to take it? What were you going to do with everything you were going to take? What would he look like? Would I be able to have a normal funeral? He walked me through them.

I finally agreed to donate Bill's organs and tissues, but I had a condition. Bill had his best friend Mark, who needed a kidney transplant, and if possible I wanted Mark to receive Bill's kidney. Unfortunately, they were not a match. I was under a lot of stress. I want you to understand that, because I tried to borrow the kidney and say, Couldn't we exchange kidneys somehow so we could get Mark a kidney? At that time, that was not proper under law. The law is a little more flexible at this point, but nonetheless that wasn't an option at the time. So I went ahead and consented.

Three tests—well, several tests had to be done, but three neurosurgeons had to certify that Bill was brain dead. Started another whole process in my mind. If he is not really dead, you are going to kill him when you take him off of oxygen for 5 minutes, and I went through the decisionmaking process all over again. I signed the papers. They went forward.

I stayed for every test except for the oxygen deprivation test, probably because I knew in my mind that he was gone and I wasn't ready to accept it at that point. They were able to take all of his organs and his tissues. They took the bones in his arms and his legs. They took the skin off of his back to use for burn victims. They took all of his organs. When the neurosurgeon summed up the results of all of the tests, he came to me and told me there was no reason this man should be dead. That didn't help, but he was gone and he wasn't coming back, and there was no reason to allow people who could use his organs not to go on living.

Bill wasn't coming back. There was no question about it. It was my ability to do something positive and take a tragedy and put a positive spin on it. I had lots of help from the Washington Regional Transplant Consortium. They have lots of grievance groups and support groups that I was able to take advantage of.

The one thing that just did it for me was when I asked the coordinator, What am I going to tell my children? I have two little boys—at that time who were 4 and 5—what am I going to tell them? And he looked me in the eye and said, You tell them that their father was a hero, he saved lives. And to this day, 13 people are alive because we gave Bill's organs and his tissues. He is a hero.

Thank you. I am available for questions.

[The prepared statement of Susan Kantrowitz follows:]

PREPARED STATEMENT OF SUSAN KANTROWITZ

Good afternoon! My name is Susan Kantrowitz, and I am representing myself as a donor family member. My husband, William Colbert, Sr., was a deceased donor. I am here to tell you my story. Thank you for this opportunity. It is indeed my pleasure.

It was an ordinary Friday night in August 1999. My mother came for dinner. My four-year-old son was bouncing off the walls as only four-year-olds can do, and my one-year-old was doing a little furniture surfing, testing his newly-acquired walking skills. My husband changed after dinner and went back to work. Bill was the Deputy Chief Counsel at the Bureau of Engraving and Printing and needed to take a deposition from a member of the night shift.

I got up with the baby around midnight and heard my husband return. He headed down to the basement to begin putting his notes together on the computer. After the baby was asleep, I decided to go down and see how Bill was doing.

I found Bill on the floor. He had laid down and put a toy under his head. It was obvious that something was wrong, and when I couldn't wake him, I called 911. I called a neighbor to come stay with the boys and started for the hospital. One of the paramedics took me aside as they were putting Bill into the ambulance. He told me it didn't look good—he pointed to his own head and implied that there was something wrong inside Bill's head.

We live less than a block from Mount Vernon Hospital and I chose to walk over. On my way, I met my neighbor. He gave me his cell phone and immediately joined me at the hospital so I wouldn't be alone. After a long wait, a nurse came in and told me they put Bill on a respirator. She explained that this was routine practice as a precaution. They also called in a neurosurgeon.

After examining my husband, the neurosurgeon called me into Bill's room. Bill had no responses. A CAT scan revealed a massive amount of blood in the brain. A blood vessel broke—there was no telling why. Bill had suffered a massive stroke and was gone. Technically he was brain dead, although his body had not died yet.

It was at that time that we started to discuss organ donation. As soon as it was mentioned, I had a flashback to an episode of the "ER" television program some years earlier. Bill and I never watched "ER," but for some reason, it was on that evening. In that episode, a teenage girl needed a lung transplant to survive. In the next room, there was a badly burned fireman who was going to die. As only Hollywood would have it, he was a perfect match for the teenage girl. In the episode, the doctors have a great debate about hastening the death of the firefighter so the transplant could be done and the teenage girl saved.

I remember it well because the next morning on our way to work. We discussed the episode. We noted how irresponsible the episode was to infer that those kinds of debates actually happen and that an individual might not be saved because he/she was an organ donor. We both felt that it was unconscionable to plant that kind of seed in the public's mind. Both of us agreed that we wouldn't hesitate to donate our organs if the opportunity presented itself. It was the right thing to do.

Even remembering this conversation, I didn't agree immediately. My husband was lying in a hospital room—for all intents and purposes alive. Yes, he was breathing with the help of the respirator, but as the nurse told me, that was routine. His kidneys were functioning, his skin was warm to the touch, and on this hot August night, he was sweating.

I sat with my brother-in-law, also a doctor. He looked at the CAT scan. He confirmed that Bill wouldn't survive. Regardless, I still had an overwhelming feeling of abandoning him. I felt that I was turning my back on him and sending him to his death. My heart and my head were telling me two different things.

The coordinator from the Washington Regional Transplant Consortium, Mr. David DeStefano, was fabulous. He sat with me and answered all of my questions. He explained that one donor can save 50 lives, not only through organs, but through tissues and bone as well. He met with me endlessly answering question after question: What would happen to the body? How would he look?

I agreed to donate Bill's organs and tissues, with one condition. Bill's best friend Mark needed a kidney. I wanted Bill's kidney to go to Mark, if they were a match. We agreed that Bill would become a deceased donor. Unfortunately, Bill and Mark were not a match. I asked if we could "barter" his kidney for another that would match Mark. The law at that time, did not allow that kind of arrangement. I went forward with the donation. It was the right thing to do.

Bill underwent a thorough examination to be sure that there was no disease or damage to the organs. Part of that was a test to ensure that Bill was in deed brain dead. Three different doctors had to certify that he would not recover from the stroke. I had another conversation with Mr. DeStefano. If there was any chance whatsoever that Bill was going to survive, I didn't want the organ donation tests to kill him. One of the tests was oxygen deprivation for five minutes. Again, I was assured that Bill was not returning. I had to trust the doctors that they were telling me the truth. I was still dealing with this tragedy. I was now a widow and my boys were fatherless.

I signed the papers allowing the doctors to take everything and anything usable. Before going into the operating room, I met with the leader of the surgical team. He cried with me as I asked that Bill be treated with the utmost dignity—as if he would survive the surgery. He assured me that they would, and I kissed him good bye as he went into surgery.

They were able to take and use all of his organs, his corneas, the skin off his back (to be bandages for burn victims) and the bones from his arms and legs. A few days after the funeral, a friend called to apologize that his wife couldn't attend the funeral with him because she was with their granddaughter who was having surgery. She was born with deformities in her leg bones and they were going to remove the affected bone and replace it with bone from a cadaver. I was able to tell my friend that I knew all about the procedure, because Bill's bone had gone to just such a bank.

In donating Bill's organs and tissues, I was able do something positive with a tragedy. I have never been sorry. The Washington Regional Transplant Consortium has been wonderful. I have been able to take advantage of numerous support groups that they sponsor, and faithfully attend the Annual Family Gathering where deceased donors are remembered and thanked. This has become crucial for my boys, who are now seven and four years old. With them, I hope to soon meet the recipients of Bill's organs and tissues. I have received tremendous support from them and am now enjoying returning the favor. I am always happy to talk on behalf of organ and tissue donation.

Before I finally decided to donate Bill's organs and tissues, I asked Mr. DeStefano about dealing with my boys. I wondered what I should tell them. He told me to tell them that their father was a hero. He said that Bill was no different from a fireman or policeman. He saved lives. He was a hero.

Thank you for your attention. I am happy to answer your questions.

Mr. GREENWOOD. We thank you for your courage today as well as on that day.

Ms. Koller.

TESTIMONY OF CHERYL KOLLER

Ms. KOLLER. Good morning. Thank you for inviting me this morning. My name is Cheryl Koller, and I am the mother of a 10-year-old little girl named Caitlyn, and Caitlyn was 8 years old when she was the recipient of a heart transplant. She had just celebrated her 8th birthday in January 2001 when she became ill with what we thought was just a stomach virus.

Caitlyn had always been a healthy and active child and there seemed to be no cause for any immediate concern. After 2 weeks of waiting for her to get better, our pediatrician sent us to the hospital to have some routine testing done. An x-ray revealed that Caitlyn's heart had enlarged and was twice the normal size and she was in heart failure. At that time, Caitlyn was transferred to the Pediatric Intensive Care Unit at the University of North Carolina's Childrens Hospital in Chapel Hill. And for 2 weeks, the doctors attempted to control the situation with medications, but they were unsuccessful.

On February 23, 2001, Caitlyn's name was placed at the top of the National Transplant List. We were told that we had the sickest child in the southeastern United States, and just a few weeks earlier she had been perfectly healthy.

This was an extremely sad time for our family. We were very afraid of the possibility of facing the future without our daughter, and there was also the confusion of her ever-changing health status, and now a desperate wait for a new heart to become available. Eight days into our wait, the doctors told us to prepare ourselves to say goodbye, because they didn't believe that Caitlyn could make it through another night. But this tough little girl did make it through that night, and 2 days later surgeons at UNC attached a ventricular assist device that was meant for adults to Caitlyn's heart, and this machine kept Caitlyn's heart pumping for the next 10 days as we continued our wait.

On the evening of March 14, my husband and I had gone to the hospital chapel to pray. We spent a lot of time praying and asking God to inspire a family faced with the death of their child, to give the gift of life to our child. It is a very difficult prayer to offer up, but we prayed with a great deal of faith and hope that God would show us His way.

When we returned to Caitlyn's room a few moments later, we were told that a heart had been found for Caitlyn. We spent a lot of time that evening praying for a very brave family that we didn't know but we owed our future happiness to.

The 8-hour transplant surgery began in the early hours of March 15. One week after the transplant, Caitlyn was taken off the ventilator. A dedicated team of doctors, nurses, and therapists were there with us to greet a little girl who was ready to live and play again.

Three days later Caitlyn stood up and took her first steps in nearly a month-and-a-half. It has now been 2 years and 3 months since Caitlyn's transplant. She went back to school full time this past school year, and she just finished the third grade. She loves to ride her bike to the playground, go swimming, and play with all the girls on our street. She has conquered a lot of obstacles, including a post-transplant stroke, to return to a fairly normal life. The doctors still cannot tell us exactly what caused Caitlyn's heart to fail, but they say she is a true miracle child.

This past February, we had the honor of meeting Phyllis and Nathan Slifer, the parents of Joseph Michael Ebert, Caitlyn's donor. And we brought a picture of Joseph with us. Joseph was a sweet, big-hearted little boy who loved life. He was 7 years old when a dirt bike accident tragically ended his life. When doctors approached Phyllis about organ donation, she said yes right away. She didn't think who would benefit. She was thinking about the son she had just lost. But something inside told her that this was the right thing to do, and she didn't want any other family to suffer the same loss that she was experiencing.

Phyllis and Nathan have found comfort in getting to know Caitlyn and us, and knowing that their son lives on through her. Joseph also lives on in a 9-year-old girl who received his liver, a 23-year-old man who received one of his kidneys, and another 7-year-old little girl who received his other kidney.

The power of one organ donor is truly amazing. One donor can potentially save 58 other lives, 8 lives through the donation of a major organ and 50 through tissue donations. And there are nearly 81,000 people waiting for an organ transplant today in the United States.

We are very fortunate that Caitlyn only waited 20 days for her transplant. A short wait is truly an exception rather than the rule.

Today I understand you will be hearing from many experts in the transplant field on ways to help increase the number of organ donations. And certainly educating Americans, the American public on organ donations will hopefully increase the number of donations and reduce the time that patients must wait for that second chance at life.

Thank you for listening to our family's story. We are truly blessed, and we are very glad that we are able to share this story with others in the hopes that it will encourage more people to give life by becoming an organ donor.

[The prepared statement of Cheryl Koller follows:]

Prepared Statement of Cheryl Koller

My name is Cheryl Koller and I am the mother of a 10 year old little girl named Caitlyn. Caitlyn was 8 years old when she was the recipient of a heart transplant.

Caitlyn had just celebrated her 8th birthday in January 2001, when she became ill with what we thought was a stomache virus. Caitlyn had always been a healthy and active child and there seemed to be no cause for any immediate concern. After two weeks of waiting for her to get better, our pediatrician sent us to the hospital to have some routine testing done. An x-ray revealed that Caitlyn's heart was twice the normal size and she was in heart failure.

Caitlyn was transferred to the pediatric intensive care unit at the University of North Carolina Children's Hospital in Chapel Hill. For two weeks the doctor's attempted to control the situation with medications but were unsuccessful. Caitlyn's name was placed at the top of the national transplant list on February 23, 2001.

This was an extremely sad time for our family. We were very afraid of the possibility of facing the future without our daughter. There was also the confusion of her ever changing health status and the desperate wait for a new heart to become available. Eight days into our wait, the doctors told us to prepare ourselves to say goodbye because they didn't believe that Caitlyn could make it through the night.

But our tough little girl did make it through that night. Two days later, surgeons at UNC attached a ventricular assist device to Caitlyn's heart. This machine kept Caitlyn's heart pumping for the next ten days as we continued our wait.

On the evening of March 14th, my husband and I had gone to the hospital chapel to pray. We'd spent a lot of time praying and asking God to inspire a family faced with the death of their child, to give the gift of life to our child. It's a very difficult prayer to offer up, but we prayed with a great deal of hope and faith that God would show us His way. When we returned to Caitlyn's room a few minutes later, we were told that a heart had been found for Caitlyn . We spent a lot of time that evening praying for a very brave family that we didn't know, but owed our future happiness to.

The eight hour transplant surgery began in the early hours of March 15th. One week after the transplant, Caitlyn was taken off the ventilator. A dedicated team of doctors, nurses and therapists were there with us to greet a little girl who was ready to live and play again. Three days later, Caitlyn stood up and took her first steps in nearly 1 1/2 months.

It's been 2 years and 3 months since Caitlyn's transplant. She went back to school full-time this past school year and has just finished the third grade. She loves to ride her bike to the playground, go swimming, and play with the girls on our street. She's conquered a lot of obstacles, including a post-transplant stroke, to return to a fairly normal life. The doctors cannot tell us exactly what caused Caitlyn's heart to fail, but they say she's a true miracle child.

This past February, we had the honor of meeting Phyllis and Nathan Slifer, the parents of Joseph Michael Ebert, Caitlyn's donor. Joseph was a sweet, big-hearted little boy who loved life. He was seven years old when a dirt bike accident tragicly ended his life. When doctors approached Phyllis about organ donation, she said yes right away. She wasn't thinking about who would benefit. She was thinking about the son she had just lost. But something inside told her this was the thing to do. She did not want any other family to suffer the same loss that she was experiencing. Phyllis and Nathan have found comfort knowing Caitlyn and knowing that their son lives on through her. Joseph also lives on in a 9-year-old girl who received his liver, a 23-year-old man who received one kidney, and a 7-year-old girl who received his other kidney.

The power of one organ donor is truly amazing. One donor can potentially save 58 other lives; eight lives through the donation of a major organ, and 50 lives through tissue donation.

There are nearly 81,000 patients waiting for an organ transplant today in the United States. A new name is added to the list every thirteen minutes. Caitlyn was very fortunate to have waited only 20 days for her new heart. A short wait is an exception rather than the rule. Seventeen people die each day waiting for a transplant.

Today you will be hearing from many experts in the transplant field on ways to help increase the number of organ donations. Educating the American public on organ donation will hopefully increase the number of organ donations and reduce the time that a patient must wait for a second chance at life. Thank you for listening to our family's story. We are truly blessed and we're glad to be able to share our story with others in the hopes that it will encourage more people to give life and become an organ donor.

Mr. GREENWOOD. Thank you, Mrs. Koller and Caitlyn.
Mr. Roth.

TESTIMONY OF JOSEPH ROTH

Mr. ROTH. Chairman Greenwood, members of the committee, subcommittee, good morning. I appreciate the opportunity to appear before you and discuss an issue that literally is life and death, that is of life-and-death importance for the tens of thousands of Americans waiting to receive organ transplants.

I am Joseph Roth, President and CEO of the New Jersey Organ and Tissue Sharing Network, the organ procurement organization serving New Jersey. I am testifying today in my capacity as the President-elect of the Association of Organ Procurement Organizations, AOPO, the organization representing all 59 federally designated OPOs in this country.

First let me say I am deeply honored to sit at the same table as such courageous people who have testified before me, and I am humbled at the honor. I applaud the subcommittee's leadership in holding today's hearing to examine how organ donation can be increased. Even though our country is blessed with the best medical technology and doctors, for a patient in need of an organ transplant, it seems almost nothing can be done to reduce the anguished wait for an organ to become to become available. Far too often time runs out before an organ can be found, if at all.

Over 80,000 people, as has been said, are waiting to receive organ transplants. While 63 people receive transplants every day, and thus a second chance at life, another 17 die on the waiting list without getting the chance, simply because not enough organs are available. The shortage of life-giving organs is a serious and chronic problem that will not be resolved without meaningful attention from policymakers.

Although there has been an increase in the number of organ donors in recent years, the rate of increase has not kept pace with the need of donated organs. Studies have found that less than 50 percent of potential eligible donors actually become donors. As a result, there is a significant potential for increased organ donation to take place and for an increased number of lives to be saved.

We simply need thoughtful policies to take advantage of this potential. No single approach is sufficient by itself to achieve large-scale increases in organ donation. The organ procurement organization community, frequently in partnership with the Department of Health and Human Services transplant-related organizations and others, instead supports a multitude of different but strategic approaches to address the national organ shortage. I would like to highlight briefly a few of them.

First, as part of a National Donation Initiative, Secretary Tommy Thompson and HHS have launched a new program to implement best practices in organ donation at the 200 hospitals with the highest potential for organ donation. The program is designed to increase organ donation rates at these hospitals to 75 percent of eligible donors. Since our national study indicates that, with some local exceptions, 80 percent of eligible donors can be found in 20 percent of the Nation's hospitals, primarily large hospitals. We believe this effort, grounded in shared accountability for organ donation needs broad-based support and we look forward to promising results from this major initiative.

Second, HHS and the Joint Commission on Accreditation of Health Care Organizations are acting on recommendations by the Secretary's Advisory Committee on Transplantation to establish policies such that a hospital's failure to identify a potential organ donor and/or refer the donor to the organ procurement organization in a timely manner, as required by law, would be considered a serious medical error. Major national meetings have been planned to address how hospitals with these missed organ donation opportunities would face appropriate review, comparable to what currently is expected for major adverse health care events.

Third, the placement of organ procurement organization staff and hospitals to be onsite organ donation coordinators is showing tremendous promise. The organ procurement organization coordinators work directly with health care professionals and families of potential donors to help them understand the importance of donation. Hospitals in which OPO coordinators are in place have experienced a significant increase in organ donation, including in inner-city settings where higher consent rates have been difficult to sustain. The Association of Organ Procurement Organization strongly endorses Federal legislation and funding to place Organ Procurement Organization coordinators in all large hospitals.

Finally, the advancement of donor rights legislation by all States is critical for giving organ donors control over their decision to donate. Eligible individuals who have declared themselves as donors deserve to have their wishes respected, with no further authorization from family members necessary. Donor rights legislation should ensure that an individual's desire to give the gift of life is carried out.

AOPO believes that advancement of this approach, with attention to public outreach, is a vital component of increased donation. We also want to assure the public that sensitivity to the needs and considerations of donors' families should not be diminished. We intend to work closely with the National Conference of Commissioners on Uniform State Laws on Donor Rights legislation and other matters of significant import, such as strengthened legislation regarding collaboration between OPOs and medical examiners and coroners.

In conclusion, policymakers and the public alike need to confront the challenge of organ shortage. Over 80,000 Americans are on the transplant waiting list. They and the thousands more who need transplants in the future deserve no less than a sustained, broad-reaching effort to increased donation. Approaches such as the ones I have described today give us hope but are useless unless they are discussed and acted upon as part of a national policy. We must work together to ensure that no one will be denied the second chance at life given by a donated organ.

Once again, thank you for the opportunity to testify today, and I will be happy to answer any questions.

[The prepared statement of Joseph Roth follows:]

PREPARED STATEMENT OF JOSEPH ROTH, PRESIDENT ELECT, ASSOCIATION OF ORGAN PROCUREMENT ORGANIZATIONS

INTRODUCTION

Chairman Greenwood and Members of the Subcommittee, I appreciate the opportunity to appear before you and discuss an issue that literally is of life and death importance for the tens of thousands of Americans waiting to receive organ transplants. I am Joseph Roth, President and CEO of the New Jersey Organ and Tissue Sharing Network, the organ procurement organization (OPO) serving New Jersey. I am testifying today in my capacity as the President Elect of the Association of Organ Procurement Organizations (AOPO), the organization representing all 59 federally-designated OPOs in the country.

PROBLEM OF ORGAN DONATION SHORTAGE

AOPO applauds the Subcommittee's leadership in holding today's hearing to examine how organ donation can be increased. Even though our country is blessed with the best medical technology and doctors, for a patient in need of an organ transplant, it seems almost nothing can be done to reduce the anguished wait for an organ to become available. Far too often, time runs out before an organ can be found, if at all. Over 80,000 people wait to receive organ transplants. While 63 people receive transplants everyday, and thus, a second chance at life, another 17 people die on the waiting list without getting that chance simply because not enough organs are available.

The shortage of life-giving organs is a serious and chronic problem that will not be resolved without meaningful attention from policymakers. Although there has been an increase in the number of organ donors in recent years, the rate of increase has not kept pace with the need for donated organs. Studies have found that less than 50 percent of potential eligible donors actually become donors. As a result, there is significant potential for increased organ donation to take place and for an increased number of lives to be saved. We simply need thoughtful policies to take advantage of this potential.

APPROACHES TO INCREASING ORGAN DONATION

No single approach is sufficient by itself to achieve large-scale increases in organ donation. The OPO community, frequently in partnership with the Department of Health and Human Services (HHS), transplant-related organizations, and others, instead supports a multitude of different but strategic approaches to address the national organ shortage. I would like briefly to highlight a few of them:

1) First, as part of a national Donation Initiative, Secretary Tommy Thompson and HHS have launched a new program to implement "best practices" in organ donation at the 200 hospitals with highest potential for organ donation. The program is designed to increase organ donation rates at these hospitals to 75% of eligible donors. Since our national study indicates that, with some local exceptions, 80 percent of eligible donors can be found in 20 percent of the nation's hospitals, primarily large hospitals, we believe that this effort grounded in shared accountability for organ donation needs broad-based support and we look forward to promising results from this major initiative.

2) Second, HHS and the Joint Commission on Accreditation of Healthcare Organizations (JCAHO) are acting on recommendations by the Secretary's Advisory Committee on Transplantation to establish policies such that a hospital's failure to identify a potential organ donor and/or refer the donor to the OPO in a timely manner—as required by law—would be considered a serious medical error. Major national meetings have been planned to address how hospitals with these "missed organ donation opportunities" would face the appropriate review, comparable to what currently is expected for major adverse healthcare events.

3) Third, the placement of OPO staff in hospitals to be onsite organ donation coordinators is showing tremendous promise. The OPO coordinators work directly with health care professionals and families of potential donors to help them understand the importance of donation. Hospitals in which OPO coordinators are in place have experienced a significant increase in organ donation, including in inner city settings where higher consent rates have been difficult to sustain. AOPO strongly endorses federal legislation and funding to place OPO organ donation coordinators in all large hospitals.

4) Finally, the advancement of Donor Rights legislation by all States is critical for giving organ donors control over their decision to donate. Eligible individuals who have declared themselves as donors deserve to have their wishes respected, with no further authorization from family members necessary. Donor Rights legislation would ensure that an individual's desire to give the "gift of life" is carried out. AOPO believes that advancement of this approach, with attention to public outreach, is a vital component of increased donation. We also want to assure the public that sensitivity to the needs and concerns of donor families should not be diminished. We intend to work closely with the National Conference of Commissioners on Uniform State Laws on donor rights legislation, and other matters of significant import, such as strengthened legislation regarding collaboration between OPOs and Medical Examiners and Coroners.

CONCLUSION

In conclusion, policymakers and the public alike need to confront the challenge of the organ shortage. Over 80,000 Americans are on the transplant waiting list. They and the thousands more who will need transplants in the future deserve no less than a sustained, broad-reaching effort to increase donation. Approaches such as the ones I have described today give us hope but are useless unless they are discussed and acted upon as part of national policy. We must work together to ensure that no one will be denied the second chance at life given by a donated organ.

Once again, thank you for the opportunity to testify today. I will be happy to answer any questions.

Mr. GREENWOOD. Thank you, Mr. Roth. And I appreciate your participation this morning. The Chair notes the presence of Mr. Tauzin, the chairman of the full committee who has joined us, and recognizes him for an opening statement.

Chairman TAUZIN. Thank you Mr. Chairman and I appreciate it. I really wanted to hear our witnesses before welcoming them because I knew their stories would be compelling, and indeed they were.

What you have assembled in this committee room today, Mr. Chairman, is an example of the courage and generosity of the organ donation story. And, Susan, your courage and the generosity of donors like Bill and others who willingly join these programs to help indeed extend the lives of our fellow citizens is not just admirable, it's amazing; and we want to thank you today for coming to share with us. I know it's difficult, extraordinarily encouraging and an uplifting story.

And we also hear of the anxiety of those who wait and who know that, you know, that organ transplants might make the difference in not only quality of life, but their life itself.

One of my staffers is an organ transplant patient who has gone through more than one transplant. She has gone through transplant rejection and transplant again and a difficult periods of complications and additional operations. I have lived this saga with her all through these various operations, and I know the anxiety she feels as she has gone through it and waited, hoped and prayed, and eventually received an organ, only to find out later on it was rejected and she had to go through the process once again.

We also have with us an example of the joy of the success stories in young Caitlyn and the extraordinary opportunities that organ donations have made in the lives of not just young people like Caitlyn but so many of our friends and relatives and fellow Americans. And so we see it all today laid before us: the courage, the generosity, the anxiety, the joy, and success.

We are also looking at three features of the organ transplant story. One we see the glorious sort of development, and that is the amazing success and advancement of science in this field, the extraordinary reach that science is extending in terms of organ transplant, capability of survival rates. The Wall Street Journal yesterday had a great story on new research and the use of anti-rejection machines that may well extend dramatically the success rates of organ transplants and therefore the lives of recipients of organ donation.

We also celebrate the glorious success stories of Caitlyn and others and we know have the benefit of that new medicine now. At the same time, we witness the tragedy of people who wait and wait, and suffer the anxiety of knowing that if only an organ donor came forward with a match, if the science advanced quick enough, that their lives might be extended.

At the same time, we also examine the promise of changes and that are going to make a difference, I think in this organ transplant story, and I hope as we hear the ongoing recommendations and the ongoing suggestions for policy changes, are going to make a difference in the success rates of the program.

I think it's important we commend Secretary Thompson at the Department of Health, who, as Governor of Wisconsin, turned his State into a model of improving rates of organ donation. He brought that same big heart, if you will, to the issue of how can we make the Nation now a model for organ transplant rates and for increasing the rates of donation throughout America. We know the recommendations of his Advisory Committee on Transplantation and we are going to hear this morning about what those recommendations consist of and how quickly can we implement.

But we will do something later on in the third panel that I wanted to highlight, and I wanted our colleagues to hear this. Not so long ago—I love "Discover" magazine, it is a great lay science journal and I read it every month when it comes out—and not so long ago, in an issue of "Discover" volume 22 number 7 July 2001, I read of a pair of brothers in Massachusetts who were doing some extraordinary work on cell regeneration and cell growth and tissue engineering. And the story in "Discover" magazine outlined how the Vacanti brothers in Massachusetts discovered spore-like cells and human mammalian tissue. That they began to work with that seemed to have potential capabilities much like stem cells; in fact, extraordinarily using these spore-like cells, they were able to build biodegradable scaffolding structures that were able to create bridges and damage tissue.

In the story—these are the guys that you might recall that built the human ear on the back of a mouse, reconstructed it. We are not just talking about organs that might save human lives, we are talking now about the possibility of using your own tissue to regenerate organs, to regenerate features of the human body that were missing or damaged, such as an ear, a damaged pancreas that might need to produce insulin, or a damaged lung that might need to be repaired. In fact, I think they took a lamb's lung, living tissue, and removed it and built the scaffolding; and with the spore cells from that lamb, rebuilt that lung tissue, according to this story, which I think is about 14 different types of cells regenerated and reconstructed. They took rats and severed their spines and regenerated in some cases a spinal connection using these spore cells.

Now, Dr. Vacanti, I think, is going to be here on the third panel, but it is going to be an amazing panel. If this is true, if this is the future of medicine, of tissue regeneration and tissue engineering, what extraordinary promise science may hold yet in terms of not only waiting for someone else to donate an organ to you but the potential or capability of your own body tissue, these spore-like cells that could be used to regenerate organs and tissues that are missing or damaged in the human body.

And so today it is a story of tragedy, but also success and glory and promise. And in structuring this subcommittee, Mr. Chairman, I want to thank you for doing it because you have laid it out for us in the future panels. And from it all I hope we can be a force as a committee to encourage the implementation of some of these ideas and the advancement of some of these technologies and to spread the hope and to spread the success stories and to cherish and celebrate the courage and the generosity of American donors, and to end the anxiety of those who wait, like Reginald, and so many others like you.

So again, Mr. Chairman, this is an extraordinary hearing you are conducting today, and I wanted to encourage you and the members of the subcommittee and the full committee to take this as a very important first step, but to walk the long mile until we fully explore all the promise that this hearing is going to lay before us.

And I thank you and yield back the balance of my time.

Mr. GREENWOOD. The Chair thanks the chairman for his statement and recognize myself for 10 minutes for questions. Let me tell you that the primary motivation for me to hold this hearing and to bring all of our witnesses today is to learn how we can expand dramatically the number of organs that are donated so that we stop what's happening in America right now, and that is 16 or 17 people dying every single day, waiting for an organ.

That's 6,000 people a year, while a number comparable to that, 6,000 people are buried or cremated with perfectly good organs that could save the other 6,000 lives but don't. So we know that so many different programs have been attempted to try to expand the number of potential donors, but with little result, frankly. The percentage of Americans who are donating organs is pretty much of a flat line.

And so I want to—I want to make sure that what happened to Caitlyn happens to Mr. Augustus. And I want to make sure that the heroism of Ms. Kantrowitz—the accent is on the first syllable, right, Kan'trowitz—is something that every American that has the opportunity makes.

And so I want to ask this question. Now, you heard in her opening statement the gentlelady from Colorado, Ms. DeGette, express in very strong terms her opposition to any financial incentive, and she correctly states that for most of our history that has been the policy of not only of the Federal Government, where it still is, but of most organizations, ethical organizations, medical organizations. That's changing. The AMA has said now that it favors at least study on what might be the impact of financial incentives.

I will tell you candidly that I don't share the gentlelady's view on this. I take the opposite view. I believe in financial incentives, that could for instance place Federal dollars into the estate of a donor, would probably serve as an incentive to get—we know that many Americans voluntarily check off the form when we renew our driver's license or in some other way we fill out an organ donor card. But many Americans, most Americans I believe, don't do that.

So the question is, would some kind of—would the notion that you can leave something a little extra in your estate for your family, should the unusual circumstance occur to you as happened to Mr. Kantrowitz, would that expand the donation rate and would that save more lives? And to me, saving an additional life or thousands of lives certainly overcomes any ethical argument that I can see for creating a financial incentive. So I just want to go down the panel and ask—I don't know if you have thought about these things—but I'd like to ask each of our witnesses whether—what your view is of that.

Ms. KOLLER. I do not believe that compensating someone for this gift should be necessary. I think that there are many Americans who are quite willing to make this gift, and I'm hoping that through more education that more Americans will be organ donors. So I don't agree with the idea of compensating.

One interesting thing, though, when my parents went to renew their licenses in Georgia, they were given a $5 discount for signing up to be an organ donor, which I thought was quite interesting. And they took it. And so maybe just something little like that could be something that, you know, we could consider just a suggestion to the States maybe, just to make people stop and think about it for a second, because I think that a lot of people do want to donate but they just don't think to do it at the time when they are renewing their licenses.

Mr. GREENWOOD. Okay. I thank you very much.

Ms. Kantrowitz.

Ms. KANTROWITZ. I'm not sure that compensation would have made a difference in whether I chose to donate Bill's organs and tissues, and I do believe that education is key here because there is so much out there that works against organ donation. However, I am open to financial compensation, and I think the key here is the type and amount of compensation you're talking about. Are you talking about giving people money? Are you talking about helping with funeral benefits? Are you talking about support and grievance help? Are you talking about help with the children afterwards? There are so many ways I think that you can do that without actually just handing people cash to make it seem—it just—actually it just seems horrible that somebody would pay me money for my liver. On the other hand, you know, there are people dying and we need to create an incentive.

So what other kinds of contributions can you make to that person? I would be in favor of looking at that. I'm not—I'm not saying that I'm not open to downright cash. I'm just saying I would like the committee to look at other ways such as I just suggested.

Mr. GREENWOOD. And if I may add, before we continue, I'm not aware that anyone has considered a cash payment to a person while they are alive. The question would be some kind of an insurance policy that would be reclaimable by the estate in the event where someone dies and their organs in fact are donated.

Mr. Augustus.

Mr. AUGUSTUS. As you mentioned before, there are some strong ethical concerns in regards to, you know, any type of financial or monetary payments to somebody or someone's family. You just have to be careful when you know you're talking about this, because this could open, you know Pandora's box, you know. To do something like that, you know, you could have, say, people out here widespread trying to, you know, if you start with—let's say there's somebody, as she mentioned before, if you just want to pay for their funeral services or give some type of benefits or some type of insurance plan, then what's going to happen after that? Someone's going to continue to try to push the envelope and, you know, then you'll have people out trying to get, you know, thousands of dollars, you know, to get the organs for people who have low income. There could be a variety of reasons.

You know, there's other countries where that does happen, where people actually sell their organs, you know, I guess on the black market. But, yeah, I have some concerns about that, you know; how would you go about doing that? I mean, that's a very slippery slope you'd slide down if you tried to do that. And that's——

Mr. GREENWOOD. Thank you, sir.

Mr. Roth.

Mr. ROTH. Mr. Chairman, the Association of Organ Procurement Organizations has said as a public policy that they would support well-controlled public demonstration projects, pilot projects, as you know. But, again, what shape those should take is really to be determined by the entire community and not just by AOPO.

Mr. GREENWOOD. Okay, thank you. In the time that remains, one of the approaches—I'd like to address this question to you, Mr. Roth. One of the approaches to increasing organ donation that you mentioned is placement of OPO organization—organ procurement organization staff in hospitals to be onsite organ donation coordinators. At the present time, how does OPO staff interact with the hospital in the organ donation process?

Mr. ROTH. Under the Federal conditions of participation, Medicare conditions of participation for organ donation, all Medicare hospitals must refer potential—well, all deaths and potential—imminent deaths to the OPO servicing them in a timely manner. An imminent death is someone who may be on a ventilator who meets certain criteria that would lead to brain death. That would allow the OPO to triage the referral and then send a staffer, someone we call a transplant coordinator, that is usually a highly trained nurse or ancillary medical professional, to go onsite to do a chart review and determine whether that potential donor could possibly become a real donor.

Of course, at that point, we interact with the staff in the hospital. Sometimes that's a very good collaborative type of system. The conditions of participation require that the hospital and the OPO work collaboratively to determine how they would approach the family for donation. Again, that doesn't work in 100 percent of the cases. It's a system that—where we spend a lot of time developing the hospitals to understand the protocol, but there's staff turnover at times, people who haven't been hit in a timely manner. But for the most part, we try to deal with a collaborative approach to the family, when brain death is declared, to offer them the option of donation at that point.

Mr. GREENWOOD. In your opening statement you said that inner-city hospitals have difficulty sustaining high consent rates for donation. Do you know why that is?

Mr. ROTH. It's a cultural issue, I believe. It's the demographics of the inner city. There are a lot of myths and misconceptions about organ donation, Mr. Chairman. For instance, there are beliefs by people that it is against their religion to donate. Well, in fact, there is no prohibition by any major religion against donation. In fact, in most religions it's considered the highest charitable act. I believe Pope John, 2 years ago, issued a statement in Rome saying that it's a Catholic's duty to become an organ donor if the option is presented to them. So it is not—there is no major religious prohibition.

There are other myths and misconceptions that are perpetrated by the media, by television, and so on, such as organs being sold for profit within the country, people being found in alleyways cut up with organs missing. Those are all myths. That's never happened in this country. But again they are perpetrated and people get scared when they have to think about the finality of their life. And that's what really I think gets to the crux of the matter. When you talk to somebody about organ donation, you're talking to them about them dying because you have to die to become an organ donor, and most of us just don't want to discuss that.

Mr. GREENWOOD. Right. Okay, thank you. My time has expired. The gentleman from Florida is recognized.

Mr. DEUTSCH. Thank you, Mr. Chairman. Thank you all for being here today and sharing your stories of pain and frustration and joy in times of bereavement. The decision of whether or not to donate a loved one's organs can indeed be a difficult and trying choice to make.

Mrs. Kantrowitz, I have to commend you for your bravery, strength, and generosity in choosing to give life to others while you yourself were forced to face the tragic loss of your husband, as well as the idea of having to live day in and day out with the knowledge that there is nothing a parent can do to help their critically ill child is a terrifying and humbling reality for many families.

Ms. Koller, I cannot tell you how happy I am to hear your daughter's good fortune, improving health as a result of a heart transplant. I wish her a full and happy life filled with many joys. Unfortunately Mrs. Koller's story of a successful transplant is not a more common occurrence today.

Mr. Augustus, I am sorry for the pain and suffering but I am nevertheless impressed and touched by your dedication to this cause and your obvious courage. I wish you the very best. I can only hope that you will be able to receive a successful kidney transplant sometime in the near future. Thank you for being here, and you know that our thoughts are with you during this difficult time.

I would like to inquire as to whether or not any of you have any recommendations about how to increase organ donations in the United States; specifically, any programs, proposals, ideas, that you have heard about or read about that are especially noteworthy or deserving of more consideration.

Ms. KOLLER. In North Carolina, we recently added a curriculum unit to the ninth and tenth grade health curriculum and so all ninth and tenth graders are introduced during a health education class to organ donation. So that's the new initiative being done in North Carolina.

Ms. KANTROWITZ. I would agree with that. I think education at an early age is very very important. When I was in the fourth grade—and we won't say how long ago that was—there were these two ugly lungs in my science class. And they were the antismoking campaign. And to this day, I can see those ugly lungs in my mind. And my parents smoked and I never did. I never did that once.

Part of the problem is that when I'm thinking about—when someone's thinking about organ donation, they are in the midst of a tragedy. I mean, their loved one is going to die; and then to be hit with "And are you ready to give up their organs?" which is not what the hospitals are necessarily saying, but that's how it appears to someone in that spot. You know, wait a minute, you're taking my husband from me and now you want his organs and tissues, too. If you're not well versed or even familiar with what goes on, it's very difficult to make those decisions.

So anything you can do, starting young, or even hitting adults to educate—you know, a public education campaign I think is only helpful because it gets people thinking. I think the gentleman is right. It has to do with thinking about your mortality. But at the same time, then, when the hospitals do come to you and say are you willing, at least you've heard of it, you understand what's going on and what's at stake. To wait till the tragedy occurs is difficult.

Mr. DEUTSCH. Mr. Augustus.

Mr. AUGUSTUS. I have to agree with these two ladies here that education, first and foremost, is probably the most important thing that we need to do. You know, get the awareness out to the community, you know. That will really help to get people to understand who are ignorant to, you know, as you mentioned before, really what organ donation is all about and the myths and things like that.

Speaking on other programs that they have, I had read some time ago about the process that she was saying before, when it wasn't an option for her husband's friend to get the organ, if you have one willing ready to give and if they have a match for him somewhere else, they could switch; which I don't see that there's anything wrong with that if there's an organ that wants to be donated, there's another organ, and this person needs this one and this person needs that one. And I saw where they have done that here, even in this area, at the Washington Hospital Center. I think it was in the Post. It was maybe over a year ago now. But they have a program, I don't know how much anyone's aware of that, where they can do that, where you can actually if you have an organ for a donation, you can get a match for someone else and they can get a match for what you need it for.

Mr. DEUTSCH. Mr. Roth.

Mr. ROTH. Thank you, Mr. Deutsch. I have laid out four issues that we support, obviously, as policy positions that should be looked at as ways to increase organ donation. And I support many of the comments made here at the table by the other witnesses.

Certainly education is important. Look at how much money has been put behind smoking and drug abuse and it's had some impact, obviously. That should happen to organ donation.

I certainly applaud Congress in the last few years for making appropriations available for grants and research into organ donation. And I say more should be done. The last appropriation for organ donation was around $10 million. When you think about that compared to organ donation—I mean to smoking and to drug abuse, antidrug abuse campaigns, it's just a drop in the bucket. We're looking at a need for a campaign that crosses generations. As was said, you have to start early to change people's ideas. With the diversity of our country, one message is not enough. We have to talk about many messages to help people understand why it is important that they become organ donors when the option is presented to them.

Mr. DEUTSCH. Thank you. Mr. Roth, in your testimony you state that your organizations supports implementation of best practices at the 200 hospitals with the highest potential for organ donation. You further state, "We believe that this effort, grounded and shared accountability for organ donation, needs broad-based support." Could you please elaborate as to exactly what those practices should be?

Mr. ROTH. Well, the interesting thing is when one examines the organ procurement organization community, you will find that there's no one best practice. When you walk into one hospital, you've only really seen one hospital. Each hospital is a culture unto itself. Each organ donation region is a region unto itself. One has to look at the uniqueness of those donors, donation service areas, to see what might work best with them.

One thing we think that has great potential across all the OPO community is the in-hospital transplant coordinator. The early data from pilot studies in several different locations have shown a substantial—a potential for substantial increase in organ donation in high-potential hospitals. We certainly support Secretary Thompson's initiative to look at best practices and work toward improving the consent rates in the 200 hospitals with the highest donation potential. That in itself could probably yield some significant results when it is fully implemented.

Mr. DEUTSCH. What department within HHS would be responsible for this implementation that you described? How do you view it?

Mr. ROTH. It's under HRSA, the Division of Transplantation.

Mr. DEUTSCH. You shared—when you spoke, you shared about the accountability within the organ donation community. I guess what I hear you saying, that there's no one successful program; that it really is multifaceted. And how do you sort of judge that in terms of evaluating those types of programs?

Mr. ROTH. Well, I mean in my service area, northern New Jersey, we have one of the most diverse populations in the country. And the messages that we have to get out to the various constituencies we deal with, from the people, you know, the citizens of that area, to the staff of the various hospitals that we serve is different for each different group. We have—we work very closely with the African American community. We work very closely with the Latino Hispanic community. We approach the Hispanic—I mean the Asian community, and each one of those takes a different message.

Yet in some areas of the country, they don't have as much of that diversity, so their approach is different as to how they address their communities. And so one has to look at how one has to focus their resources. And our resources obviously are limited so as a not-for-profit agency, you know, there's just so much we can put behind donor enhancement education efforts.

Mr. DEUTSCH. You state in your testimony that you believe on-site donation coordinators show tremendous promise. Is funding the major impediment to deploying OPO coordinators in all large hospitals? And also has HHS been receptive and supportive of that proposal?

Mr. ROTH. The answer to the first question is funding, yes, is crucial to this project. And yet—and the second question is, yes, HHS has been supportive. The results of the pilot studies are as a result of a Division of Transplantation grant to look into that.

So the thing about in-house coordinators, Mr. Deutsch, is that studies have shown that there are several things that impact the immediate donation situation. One of them, obviously, is recognizing the potential donor in a timely manner. Things happen out in the system. The trauma departments change the way they address patients that are brought in with a traumatic injury. One of the things we're seeing in our service areas is that the trauma departments are moving toward earlier asking of families for a "do not resuscitate" or DNR order, which they then implement as a do not treat. So by the time we get onsite, the potential donor may not be as viable for donation as we would like them to be. So we're actually moving to get onsite earlier, before this discussion goes into place.

But there are other issues that go on. A lot of it is how the family is treated when they go onsite for their loved one's crisis. Here is a family in crisis. And a lot of them walk into the hospital, and nobody's paying attention to them. Now, it's not because they're deliberately not paying attention to them; it's because if you walk into a trauma unit that's very busy, people are running around trying to save lives. So having an in-hospital coordinator onsite who can address the needs of the family during their time of crisis can hopefully predispose them toward donation.

Mr. DEUTSCH. If I can just ask for unanimous consent that the ranking Democrat on the full committee's statement be entered into the record.

Mr. GREENWOOD. Without objection, it shall be.

The gentleman from Oregon is recognized for 10 minutes.

Mr. WALDEN. Thank you, Mr. Chairman. I don't have a lot of questions, but I guess just a reflection on some of the comments, and I appreciate your testimony.

I think for a lot of people when they think about organ donation, what happens to a loved one, you almost in your mind conjure up a picture of Frankenstein and pieces being put together, and so I think your comments about the need for early education are extraordinarily important so people understand early on in the process just what's involved at a young stage in their lives, so it just becomes a natural thing to do. And certainly the more we can facilitate the decision way ahead of time, the better.

And that's where these license—driver's license programs make a lot of sense. And I wonder, too, about any work that's being done with health insurance companies. It seems to me—or life insurance companies—that as you go through those processes, signing up for life insurance or health insurance, that maybe there's another opportunity to network and make this opportunity available and work on the education point.

Mr. Roth, or any of you, would like to respond?

Mr. ROTH. If I might just, you know, Secretary Thompson has implemented the Business Partnership for Donation in which they are recruiting corporations, working with the organ procurement community and transplant community, to recruit businesses all across the country to implement organ donation. So your question, Mr. Walden, actually goes much further, where you're taking it past the insurance companies to major corporations, small businesses and so on, to where you can implement programs to talk up donation amongst the employees of that business.

Mr. WALDEN. But do you know on the issue of health insurance and life insurance——

Mr. ROTH. On the insurance, no, there is nothing that I am aware of at this moment.

Mr. WALDEN. Is there a check-off that we can encourage?

Mr. ROTH. No, I'm not aware of that at the moment.

Mr. WALDEN. At least when you sign up for your driver's license in a State like Oregon, you get that option. You make a decision. And I just wonder if that might be another way to get people to make that decision.

Mr. ROTH. That's certainly worth discussing.

Mr. WALDEN. Does anyone else have a comment along those lines?

Then the other issue I have is just if you could speak to the issue of the advancement in immunosuppressant drugs and how this is evolving, and I'd be curious from a firsthand status to OPO.

Ms. KOLLER. Caitlyn is doing very well on her immunosuppressants. Over the last 2 years they have been able to go lower and lower so that she's on very few drugs at this time. But of course, we're always interested in what the drug companies are, you know, researching in hopes that they can get her on a drug with the least amount of side effects as possible. But we have been very fortunate. There's very few signs of rejection, so she's doing very well on her immunosuppressants.

Mr. WALDEN. And what about cost and coverage? Does your insurance——

Ms. KOLLER. Once again we are very fortunate, because her immunosuppressants would cost us well over $1,000 a month, probably closer to $2,000 a month. And because of our copay situation, I would say that her monthly cost of medications may be about $60. But we are blessed to be under a very good insurance program. Our benefits will go up to $2 million, I believe, for her.

Mr. WALDEN. You're worried about the cap.

Ms. KOLLER. Right. And the insurance company has assured us it takes a long time to rack up bills of $2 million. So—but I know that we're probably halfway there, at least to the million dollar mark, because just the whole cost of being in an intensive care unit for so long and a rehab hospital. So at some point we may be, you know, forced with the decision of how are we going to pay for drugs, especially if we hit that cap at any time.

Mr. WALDEN. Right. Okay. Any other comments? Mr. Augustus.

Mr. AUGUSTUS. When I first got set up——

Mr. GREENWOOD. Go ahead and pull it right up to you.

Mr. AUGUSTUS. When I first got set up at the Washington Hospital Center a couple of years ago on the transplant list, I went through a process where I spoke with the social worker, transplant coordinator, the surgeon. We went through a whole list of people and they explained that process. And it is quite expensive for the immune suppressant drugs. But they've—from what they've told us and what, you know, I've learned is that they've come a long way, finding out what works best, they adjust them depending on the person's body and how they affect them. They try to get down to the lowest dosage as possible. But it is expensive.

And for a person who is on dialysis, such as myself, under 55 you can get Medicare, which I do have as my secondary coverage and I believe that they pay, they told me, about 80 percent of those immune suppressant drugs. But I believe that currently, after 36 months after a transplant or if you come off dialysis or anything, the Medicare will be gone if you're under 55. So that is a concern because they are expensive. But I think they're trying to pass legislation now to get it for, you know, for a lifetime. But I don't know right now what the current status is, but I know about a year and a half ago they just got it where certain people who met certain criteria could get it for a lifetime. But I don't fall under that category at this time. But they're working to try to get that.

Mr. ROTH. Mr. Walden, I'm not a physician so I can't comment on the medical aspects of immunosuppression. I can echo what I do know about the cost. Certainly a lot of tremendous progress is being made daily in the development of new immunosuppressants therapies: Witness the article in yesterday's Wall Street Journal. And having worked in the pharmaceutical industry for 20 years before I entered this field, I do know that they are working at it.

Certainly there are going to be a lot of breakthroughs in the next 10 to 20 years. But as Mr. Augustus pointed out, the cost of immunosuppressant therapy is certainly a substantial issue for people waiting for transplant and people that receive transplant.

There have been some improvements in the coverage for the safety net for people who don't have the insurance coverage, but I'm not sure it's enough. And in the context of today's debate about outpatient Medicare drug coverage, this will get, you know—this is subservient to that coverage. But I do believe that if a person—if the country is willing to pay to have a person transplanted, there's got to be a way to cover them to maintain the integrity of that organ for the life of that organ as opposed to telling them that there's going to be a cutoff after 36 months if they don't have a sufficient drug coverage for that.

Mr. WALDEN. Okay. Thank you.

Mr. GREENWOOD. Would the gentleman yield?

Mr. WALDEN. Absolutely.

Mr. GREENWOOD. I just wanted to ask, Mr. Roth, are you aware of individuals in this country who either don't get transplants or don't gain—have continued access to the anti——

Mr. ROTH. Immunosuppressants.

Mr. GREENWOOD. [continuing] immunosuppressant drugs for lack of insurance and for lack of funds?

Mr. ROTH. I am not immediately aware of anybody. There have been stories of people who have had to have fundraising campaigns to pay for transplants and so on. I personally am not aware of that. And I'm personally—I have heard stories that, again anecdotally, about patients who have had to stay on disability—who could be leading a productive life—but if they stayed on disability, they will get their drugs through some program or another. And the shame of it is, is here are some people who could be productive in America, make money, pay taxes, help pay for their costs, but have to stay on disability so they can get their immunosuppressive therapy.

Mr. GREENWOOD. Ms. DeGette and I were having a side-bar conversation a little earlier about the financial issues, and it seems to me that this country spends an enormous amount of money on dialysis that goes on for years and years and years. We spend an enormous amount of money through Federal health programs, as does the private sector, on people who are patients in hospitals only because they are waiting for organs so that they can leave. So it seems to me that the cost/benefit analysis goes—always is improved by having the donation available and having that transplantation occur, not only talking about the measures of living and extending lives and so forth; but from a pure dollar-and-cent perspective, I think it makes sense to do everything we can to get the organ donations going.

The gentlelady from Colorado is recognized for 10 minutes.

Ms. DEGETTE. Thank you, Mr. Chairman. And I agree. As I mentioned, I'm the co-chair of the Diabetes Caucus, and as well as kidney transplants—it occurred to me when Mr. Tauzin was speaking about the tremendous potential of islet cell transplantation in actually curing diabetes and how critical pancreatic organ donation is for diabetes research. And as the chairman says, if we can increase islet cell transplantation and refine it, the hundreds of millions of dollars that would be saved every year in diabetes treatments will be significant—not to mention the increase in the quality of life.

I want to add my thanks particularly to these three witnesses at this end of the table for coming. I was mentioning to counsel that I think your testimony has been some of the most compelling and poised testimony that we've heard in this committee for many years. So I want to thank all of you for your perspectives. It never hits home harder than when you hear people's personal stories of what they live with every day.

And, Ms. Kantrowitz, in particular, I want to say how sorry I am for your loss and how courageous you are to be raising these boys by yourself now. But it must give you some comfort in knowing that 13 lives have been saved.

I wanted to ask you, Mr. Roth, about a couple of things. As I said, I've been interested in pediatric transplantation for a number of years and have passed legislation. When Ms. Koller was testifying about how Caitlyn was at the top of the list for heart transplants, I don't think a lot of people intuitively realized what I learned a few years ago, which is that pediatric organs can be used in adults but adult organs cannot be used in children. Yet for many years, what happened on organ donation lists was everybody would just be placed on the list, irrespective of age. And if your name came up first, then you would get the transplant, whether or not it was—in other words, adults were getting pediatric organs when there were very sick children like Caitlyn on the list. And to add to that problem, with many diseases, adults that might have—liver disease is an example. Adults that might have those diseases would be able to sustain life through treatments or dialysis for much longer than kids with pediatric diseases.

And so what my legislation was aimed to do and what I've heard anecdotally from different folks involved, is it was aimed to give— it seems so simple but yet it wasn't happening—is kids would have preferential treatment on organ donation lists for pediatric organs.

I'm wondering if you can tell me what the status of that is right now through the different organ networks. And is that happening?

Mr. ROTH. Yes, Ms. DeGette, and I'm sure that Dr. Metzger and the follow-on panel could address that in more detail.

Ms. DEGETTE. I'm planning to ask him.

Mr. ROTH. But there have been some substantial changes made to the allocation paradigms to try and give preference to pediatric recipients.

Ms. DeGETTE. And has that been done on a voluntary basis?

Mr. ROTH. It was done through the UNOS policymaking procedure.

Ms. DeGETTE. Great. Thank you. And has that helped kids get access to pediatric organs?

Mr. ROTH. I don't have the figures.

Ms. DeGETTE. Well, I'll ask him. A second thing I wanted to ask you, because you testified about donor rights legislation——

Mr. ROTH. Yes.

Ms. DeGETTE. And that seems to me to be a big issue. Listening to Ms. Kantrowitz talk about the very difficult decisions—here you are and your loved one is unexpectedly dying before you, but yet they are alive. You know they can be kept alive, and how hard it is—you know, I don't think we should infer bad motives to the family members, but you know they've got someone and they're essentially brain dead, but they can see them breathing or perspiring or whatever.

I'm wondering what the status of donor rights legislation is, because that seems to me to be something that would really not just help increase the percentage of organ donations, but increase the level of comfort for the families as they're sitting there in this very difficult situation.

Mr. ROTH. Right now I believe there are 19 States that have donor rights legislation in some form or another, including my State, New Jersey. I think there are several issues still that attend to donor rights legislation. First and foremost, the law does make the donor's decision inviolable, so that if they legally executed an organ donor card, an advance directive, a living will, that says they wish to be a donor, their family cannot—and a majority of their family cannot deny that donation.

Where we find the difficulty in implementing those laws is in finding out if those wishes have been made. There are donor registries, but they don't—they aren't sufficiently large enough yet to catch everybody that could possibly have donated. There have been attempts to make living will registries and so on.

There are other potential issues which have not been broached as yet as, you know, the scenario where a family objects so strongly that the hospital staff will not assist the organ procurement organization in recovering the organs. That has not happened, but that is certainly something that's out there to discuss about this. And if the family does not wish to move ahead with the donation, we would have some problem because we have to go to the family to ask for a medical social history so that we can have the appropriate information.

Yet I do believe, and as we state in our publicity, the Coalition on Donation, you know: Share your wishes, share your life. Not only should a person sign an organ donor card, become a willing organ donor, but make it known very strongly to their family members. Many times a patient is brought in in a traumatic injury to a hospital, and we can't find a document of gift because it was left at home or something like that. And if the family is not sure what the donor's wishes are, many times the default answer is no, just because they're not sure what that——

Ms. DeGette. And I assume folks are exploring better registries, better ways to give.

Mr. Roth. Yes. The HHS has looked at that. There has been a consensus on that.

Ms. DeGette. A second question I have is, you mentioned that many people assumed that there are religious reasons for not donating. Has your organization or other organizations made an effort through churches to educate? Can you talk for just a moment about that?

Mr. Roth. Yes. Certainly every organ procurement organization in the country has some outreach program to clergy within their service area. There is a national donor Sabbath in November, which all organ procurement organizations make a concerted effort to have clergy speak from the pulpit during that Sabbath to talk about organ donation. But clearly, having councils or task forces or advisory committees involving churches is an important part of an organ procurement organization's public education.

Ms. DeGette. I was just thinking, for example, in Denver our Black Ministerial Alliance sponsors Diabetes Day at the black churches at all the Baptist churches and some others, and they have diabetes educators and others. I would think we could even ratchet the organ transplantation and donation up a notch, you know, and have people really preaching from the pulpit on this especially, as we were discussing, in urban communities where donation rates are lower but the need is higher.

Mr. Roth. Well, Ms. DeGette, as you're pointing out, it is a question of just having many voices out there talking about organ donation.

Ms. DeGette. Yes. And my last question to you is do you know about any efforts for, say, public service advertising on television and radio outlets?

Mr. Roth. I know that, again, as part of our public relations campaigns, most OPOs do get public service advertising in outlets all around the country.

Ms. DeGette. Do you know what the level of that is at all?

Mr. Roth. I can't give you any numbers on that at all. I am just not aware of what the numbers are.

Ms. DeGette. Is that information out there? We could obtain that? The lady behind you is shaking her head yes.

Mr. Roth. Yes, I believe that information is out there.

Ms. DeGette. Mr. Chairman.

Mr. Greenwood. She's testifying next.

Ms. DeGette. Oh, she's testifying next. Good. I'll ask her then. Thank you very much and I will yield back the balance of my time.

Mr. Greenwood. The Chair thanks the gentlelady. The Chair thanks our witnesses for your courage in being here this morning and for your advising this committee. You are excused.

And we'll call forth our next panel which consists of Ms. Michelle Snyder, who is the Director of the Office of Special Programs, Health Resources and Services Administration, HRSA; and Dr. Robert Metzger, M.D., President-elect of the United Network for Organ Sharing. We welcome both of you. Thank you for being here.

As you know, this is an investigative hearing and it's our practice to take our testimony here under oath. Do either of you have any objections to giving your testimony under oath? Seeing no objection, I should advise you that you have the right to be represented by counsel pursuant to the rules of the House. Do either of you wish to be represented by counsel? Okay. In that case, if you would stand and raise your right hands.

[Witnesses sworn.]

Mr. GREENWOOD. I think we need to ask the gentleman to my left to identify himself.

Mr. ARONOFF. Yes. My name is Remy Aronoff, and I am with Michelle Snyder.

Mr. GREENWOOD. Okay. All right.

Ms. Snyder, you are recognized for an opening statement.

TESTIMONY OF MICHELLE SNYDER, DIRECTOR, OFFICE OF SPECIAL PROGRAMS, HEALTH RESOURCES AND SERVICES ADMINISTRATION; REMY ARNOFF, DEPUTY DIRECTOR; AND ROBERT METZGER, PRESIDENT-ELECT, UNITED NETWORK FOR ORGAN SHARING

Ms. SNYDER. Thank you. Good morning, Mr. Chairman and members of the subcommittee. My name is Michelle Snyder and I am the very newly appointed Director of the Office of Special Programs within the Health Resources and Services Administration. Accompanying me today is Mr. Remy Aronoff who is the Deputy Director of the Office of Special Programs, who will assist me in answering any questions that you may have.

We are pleased to appear before you——

Mr. GREENWOOD. I believe you've been on board about 3 weeks now.

Dr. SNYDER. Well actually 2. I took a week off.

Mr. GREENWOOD. Welcome.

Ms. SNYDER. We are pleased to appear before you today to discuss organ transplantation and donation, a topic that is one of Secretary Thompson's highest priorities. In fact, I think it is safe to say that the Secretary is passionate about increasing organ donation and transplantation, the true gift of life.

We have seen many recent examples of the selfless giving of individuals from many walks of life in our country. Some of the most selfless and unheralded people are those who sign organ donor cards and share their decision with their families and loved ones, families who decide to donate the organs of a loved one who has just died, and living donors who agree to share a kidney or part of a liver or bone marrow.

I am proud that many important efforts in organ donation and transplantation reside in my agency, the Health Resources and Services Administration. On October 19, 1984, when President Reagan signed into law the National Organ Transplant Act, he said, I believe that that act strikes a proper balance between private and public sector efforts to promote organ transplantation.

Almost 20 years later, that private/public relationship is a productive one. HRSA's Division of Transplantation oversees the contract held by UNOS, the United Network for Organ Sharing that runs the Organ Procurement and Transplantation Network, or

OPTN. The OPTN, whose numbers include the professionals involved in the donation and transplantation system, maintains the organ wait list and matches patients to donor organs 24 hours a day, 365 days a year.

Today there are over 80,000 people awaiting an organ. We estimate that 17 people die each day while waiting for an organ. We need to close the gap between the number of people needing organs and the number of organs available. We and our transplant community partners are currently involved in a couple of activities that are intended to increase organ donation and improve the transplantation system. I'd like to mention some of them briefly and refer you to my written testimony for details.

The Workplace Partnership for Life, which is part of Secretary Thompson's Gift of Life Donation Initiative, reaches out to people in their workplaces to increase awareness of the needs for organs. So far, over 7,000 businesses of all sorts have signed on to this program.

Another element in the Secretary's Gift of Life Initiative is the Best Practices Initiative. We have found that 50 percent of potential organs come from 200 of the largest hospitals. Therefore, we are working to identify and then to replicate the practices that lead to high donation rates in these hospitals.

Secretary Thompson, on April 25, announced our goal of raising the average rates of donation in the Nation's 200 largest donation potential hospitals to 75 percent from the current rate of 46 percent. Some hospitals and organ procurement organizations are already exceeding this goal so we know that it's possible. The Advisory Committee on Organ Transplantation, a group of 34 nongovernment organ transplantation experts from many different fields, sent 18 recommendations intended to improve the transplantation system to the Secretary last November. The Secretary reported 2 weeks ago at the most recent ACOT meeting held here in Washington that he supports all of these recommendations in principle and is committed to working with the committee.

Finally, HRSA's Division of Transplantation supports two extramural grant programs designed to increase the number of donors and donor organs available for transplant: clinical interventions to increase organ procurement and social and behavioral interventions to increase organ and tissue donation. The results from some of these projects have been received and are being replicated. We expect to receive more results and share more ways to increase organ donation in the coming months.

Next year we celebrate the 50th anniversary of organ transplantation in the United States. The first organ transplant took place in Boston in 1954. A kidney was successfully transplanted from a donor to his identical twin brother. This field of organ transplantation has come a long way from this beginning 50 years ago. My hope is that the life-giving endeavor of organ transplantation will grow even more, and that there will come a time when every American in need of a new organ will be provided one. HRSA is committed to this ambitious goal. We will do everything in our power to achieve it.

I was much struck at the recent ACOT meeting when Dr. Phil Berry, who received a new liver 16 years ago, said that the great miracle of transplantation is that you can be so sick and then you can be so well. We want this miracle to be available for each patient who can benefit from a transplant.

Thank you for your support and your efforts to increase organ donation and transplantation. And we look forward to continuing to work with you on this important issue, and we would be happy to answer any questions that you might have.

And I also have to add—I do have to do a brief commercial. For anyone in the room, on the back table there are organ donation cards, and we would be very happy for anyone to pick those up. Thank you.

[The prepared statement of Michelle Snyder follows:]

PREPARED STATEMENT OF MICHELLE SNYDER, DIRECTOR, OFFICE OF SPECIAL PROGRAMS, HEALTH RESOURCES AND SERVICES ADMINISTRATION

Mr. Chairman and Members of the Subcommittee: My name is Michelle Snyder. I am the newly appointed Director of the Office of Special Programs within the Health Resources and Services Administration. I would also like to introduce Mr. Remy Aronoff, Deputy Director of the Office of Special Programs, who will assist me in answering any questions that you may have. We are pleased to appear before you today to discuss organ donation and transplantation, a topic that is one of Secretary Thompson's highest priorities. In fact, the Secretary is passionate about increasing organ donation and transplantation—the true gift of life. Thank you for all of your efforts to increase organ donation. We look forward to continuing to work with you on this important issue.

We have seen many recent examples of the selfless giving of individuals from many walks of life in our country. Some of the most selfless and unheralded people are those who sign organ donor cards and share their decision with their families and loved ones, families who decide to donate the organs of a loved one who has just died, and living donors who agree to share a kidney or part of a liver or bone marrow. I am proud that many important efforts in organ donation and transplantation reside in my agency, the Health Resources and Services Administration.

On October 19, 1984, when President Reagan signed into law the National Organ Transplant Act, he said, "I believe that this act strikes a proper balance between private and public sector efforts to promote organ transplantation." Almost 20 years later, we still believe that. HRSA's Division of Transplantation oversees the contract held by UNOS, the United Network for Organ Sharing, that runs the Organ Procurement and Transplantation Network or OPTN. The OPTN, whose members include the professionals involved in the donation and transplantation system, maintains the organ wait list and matches patients to donor organs 24 hours a day, 365 days a year. It is dedicated to increasing the equity, effectiveness and efficiency of organ sharing through our national system of organ allocation and to increasing the supply of donated organs.

In 1992, 14,000 organs were transplanted. Ten years later, in 2002, almost 25,000 organs were transplanted. There has been progress. But at the same time, we are all sadly aware that more needs to be accomplished. At the end of 1992, 27,630 patients were awaiting an organ. Today, over 80,000 people are on the waiting list in need of an organ. Because of this shortage of organs, we estimate that each day 17 people die waiting for an organ. We and our transplant community partners are always seeking ways to improve the process of organ donation and transplantation and reduce this number of needless deaths. I'd like to tell you about some of the positive things that are currently happening.

One initiative that I am especially excited about is something we call the "Workplace Partnership for Life," which is part of Secretary Thompson's Gift of Life Donation Initiative. The Workplace Partnership for Life began about two years ago. The idea is to invite employers and employees through their workplaces to sign up as partners to create a donation friendly workplace. The workplace is a great environment in which to create awareness of the need for donation. We are inviting corporations and unions, small businesses, associations, government agencies, schools, and volunteer organizations to join the campaign. As of May 15th, 7,334 organizations across the country had joined our Workplace Partnership. The organizations represent the diversity of America—from A.G. Edwards and Sons of Virginia to the 7 O'Clock Barbershop, Incorporated, to the National Republican Legislators Association to the National Benevolent and Protective Order of Elks. These groups are educating their members and employees through newsletters, and at health and wellness fairs. Fax cover sheets include organ donation slogans. Posters are displayed by elevators. All in support of organ donation. At the end of 2002, General Motors/UAW and Blue Cross/Blue Shield of Tennessee reported more than 6,000 individuals signed-up to be donors. We estimate that our Workplace Partners at this time can reach 50 million Americans. The Secretary issued a challenge this past April for the Partners, in the coming year, to generate and document at least 1 million new people who have committed to organ donation.

On April 25, Secretary Thompson announced the newest element of his Gift of Life Initiative: A Best Practices Initiative on organ donor consent. Specifically, the Secretary announced our goal of improving donor protocols and donor management to raise the average rate of donation in the nation's 200 largest donor-potential hospitals to 75% from the current rate of 46%. We believe this is possible because some hospitals and Organ Procurement Organizations or OPOs are already exceeding this goal! We have chosen to focus on these largest hospitals because 50 percent of all potential donors are in these largest hospitals. Thus, we have the potential to save or enhance thousands of lives each year by achieving this goal. The major organizations of the donation and transplant community have joined the Secretary in this effort and we are already working together to pursue it.

We are working together to identify the best practices of high performing areas and will then assist other large hospitals and OPOs to systematically replicate these best practices, thereby increasing donation rates in these large donor-potential hospitals. We are using the collaborative method of the Institute for Healthcare Improvement, which has been successfully used to achieve dramatic improvements in hospital efficiency, clinical outcomes, and other activities in hospitals across the country.

Another important part of improving our organ transplantation system is the Secretary's Advisory Committee on Organ Transplantation. There are 34 members on the ACOT, all non-governmental experts and professionals who come from fields such as health care public policy, transplantation medicine and surgery, critical care medicine, other medical specialties, and non-physician transplant professions. They have expertise in areas such as surgery, nursing, epidemiology, immunology, law and bioethics, behavioral sciences, economics, and statistics. The Committee also has representatives of transplant candidates, transplant recipients, organ donors, and family members. It meets twice a year.

The ACOT is charged with grappling with the serious issues that affect both recipients and donors. At last November's meeting the Committee made 18 recommendations to improve our organ transplantation system. Just two weeks ago our Advisory Committee met again here in Washington. When we opened this meeting our first task was to immediately address the Committee's recommendations from the November meeting. It was with a great sense of pride and teamwork that it was announced that Secretary Thompson had agreed in principle with all of the recommendations; in fact, we have already begun implementation of most of those recommendations. Let me highlight some notable examples:

Of special emphasis were issues relating to living donation. One recommendation said that each living donor should have an independent donor advocate to ensure that informed consent standards and ethical principles are applied to the practice of all live organ donor transplantation. The Secretary fully supports this concept.

It was also recommended that the Secretary of HHS, in concert with the Secretary of Education, should recommend to states that organ and tissue donation be included in core curricula of professional schools, including schools of education, schools of medicine, schools of nursing, schools of law, schools of public health, schools of social work and of pharmacy. The Secretary has announced that he is collaborating with the Secretary of Education to develop model curriculum for use in our schools. They will be sending a joint letter to the nation's school systems to encourage them to adopt these modules in their curriculum.

In addition, as part of the Secretary's Education Initiative, Secretary Thompson and Secretary Paige will launch three projects for children and young adults from ages 10 to 22:

(1) "Decision: Donation" is a model donation program for high school students, which will be launched this summer; it focuses on high school students in health education and driver's education classes, includes hard copy, videos, CDs, and will be on-line.

(2) Internet-based learning tool, "Sandrine's Gift," is aimed at both middle and high school students. It's available on an international Internet-based education site, and has the potential to reach children around the world. It includes discussions between students in classrooms and other students who have experienced donation/transplantation themselves or in their families.

(3) The "College Donor Awareness Project" is a "tool kit" for college students to use to conduct campaigns and presentations in order to explain the critical need for organ, tissue, marrow, and blood donation.

Another Committee recommendation I want to mention concerns the concept of encouraging state legislative practices that promote increased donation and transplantation. We are in the process of identifying model state legislation that promotes donation and transplantation. Examples of productive state legislation include the Michigan and Illinois state-wide registries of donors, Arizona's and Florida's requirement to follow donor wishes for donation, and the Texas and New Jersey laws requiring medical examiners not to withhold life saving organs. We will be raising these actions to the attention of all states as model practices.

I would like to share with you one final aspect of our efforts to increase donation and transplantation. Our Division of Transplantation supports two extramural grant programs designed to increase the number of donors and donor organs available for transplant: Clinical Interventions to Increase Organ Procurement; and Social and Behavioral Interventions to Increase Organ and Tissue Donation. Five grantees are currently testing and evaluating medical techniques at hospitals and other health care facilities capable of increasing the number of possible organ donors and the number of transplantable organs. Eleven grantees are testing the success of outreach efforts and education campaigns in increasing donation rates. The results of some of these grants are already being replicated in some high-performing OPOs and hospitals. We look forward to having the results of other research efforts in and replicating positive results elsewhere in the next 3 to 5 years.

Next year, we celebrate the 50th anniversary of organ transplantation in the United States. The first organ transplant took place in Boston in 1954. A kidney was successfully transplanted from a donor to his identical twin brother. The recipient has since died from causes unrelated to the transplant. His brother, the donor, is still alive. The field of organ transplantation has come a long way from this humble beginning 50 years ago. My hope is that the life-giving endeavor of organ transplantation will prosper even more and that there will come a time when every American in need of a new organ will be provided one. HRSA is committed to this high goal. We will do everything in our power to achieve it. At the recent ACOT meeting, Dr. Phil Berry, who received a new liver 16 years ago, said that the great miracle of transplantation is that you can be so sick and then you can be so well. We want this miracle to be available for each patient who can benefit from a transplant. I look forward to working with you and am happy to answer any questions you have.

Mr. GREENWOOD. We thank you. Thank you very much.
Dr. Metzger.

TESTIMONY OF ROBERT METZGER

Mr. METZGER. Chairman Greenwood and members of the subcommittee, I appreciate the opportunity to appear before you to discuss new initiatives for increasing organ donation. I'm Dr. Robert Metzger, transplant physician and medical director of the Organ Procurement Organization and Kidney Transplant Program at Florida Hospital in Orlando. I am testifying today in my capacity as the incoming Vice President, President-elect of UNOS, United Network for Organ Sharing, the organization contracted to manage the Organ Procurement and Transplantation Network.

Over 81,000 patients are on the wait list for transplantation in the United States today, and more than 5,000 will die this year without receiving a transplant. More startling is that almost 60 percent of those on the list today will die without receiving a transplant. Yet organs from deceased donors are recovered from less than 50 percent of actual potential donors, resulting in the loss of thousands of lifesaving transplants.

Most of the small annual 1 to 2 percent increase in the number of deceased donors has come from expanding the medical and social conditions previously used to eliminate potential donors, while the wait list continues to grow at a rate of 12 percent annually.

In late April, UNOS sponsored a national consensus conference, "Maximizing the Consent Process from Research to Practice" in Orlando, Florida. Over 100 experts from the organ procurement and transplant community came together to address best practices for (1) training and maintaining recovery coordinators; (2) improving the consent process; (3) supporting the needs of donor families; and (4) evaluating the impact of "first person consent" or "donor authorization." the recommendations from the work groups will soon be published, and I will limit my discussion to those from the Work Group on Donor Authorization, moderated by Helen Leslie, Executive Director of LifeNet OPO in Virginia and myself.

In 1968 the National Conference on Commissioners for Uniform State Laws drafted the Uniform Anatomical Gift Act, the UAGA, that authorized anyone 18 years of age or more to gift any part of his body, to take effect upon death, and that this could not be rescinded without his consent by anyone. Over the next decade this was adopted by the legislature of all 50 States. However, this has been virtually ignored by all OPOs because of the small numbers of potential donors with legal donor documents and the difficulty in documenting their existence at the time of death.

In 1995 the Center for Organ Recovery and Education, or CORE, the OPO for western Pennsylvania and part of West Virginia, began accepting the donor document as legally binding. In the subsequent 7 years, they found that donation occurred 100 percent of the time when the donor document was available, but only the usual 51 percent where consent from the family was utilized.

Our work group's recommendation was to develop an aggressive national effort to increase recovery of donor organs by moving to an emphasis on the donor authorization process.

The work group then developed the following position:

One, the decedent's right to donate should take precedence in the donation process.

Two, this should be accomplished in the framework of honoring the donor's wishes, respecting the needs of recipients, and continuing to support and care for the donor family.

Three, the approach should provide a consistent level of support for the donor family; sensitivity to the needs of diverse populations; and the achievement of an effective paradigm shift by hospital staff and donation specialists in he process of recovering organs.

An action agenda was developed to create national synergy and momentum to enlist a broad-based coalition within the procurement and transplant arena and government agencies; to seek allies from the general public and greater health care community; explore the need for UAGA revisions; advance a supportive public relations strategy; and to pursue donor rights legislation in all 50 States. Also, promote donor registries as a vehicle for perhaps a national donor card and depository, and to develop multiple online access sites.

One of the problems is that a lot of us when we go to the Motor Vehicle Administration are not even old enough to sign a donor card. And in Florida, don't think you have to go back for another 6 years; and in Arizona I think it's 15 years. So you're not given the opportunity to do that license—driver's license event.

I'm happy to report that in the short month following the conference, this proposal has been endorsed by the Executive Committee of the Association of Organ Procurement Organizations, the Advisory Committee on Organ Transplantation to the Secretary of Health and Human Services, ACOT; was just this week, at the American Transplant Congress, endorsed by both the American Society of Transplantation and the American Society of Transplant Surgeons; and is under discussion by the National Kidney Foundation and the Coalition on Donation.

I am hopeful that over the next 2 years this program could result in a significant increase in the number of our citizens willing to come forward in authorizing their gift of life to their fellow citizens in need.

Thank you, and I will be willing to answer any questions.

[The prepared statement of Robert Metzger follows:]

PREPARED STATEMENT OF ROBERT METZGER, PRESIDENT-ELECT, UNITED NETWORK FOR ORGAN SHARING

INTRODUCTION

Chairman Greenwood and members of the Subcommittee, I appreciate the opportunity to appear before you to discuss new initiatives for increasing organ donation. I am Dr. Robert Metzger, a transplant physician and Medical Director of the Organ Procurement Organization and kidney transplant program at Florida Hospital in Orlando. I am testifying today in my capacity as the in-coming Vice President/President-Elect of UNOS, the United Network for Organ Sharing, the organization contracted to manage the Organ Procurement and Transplantation Network.

ORGAN DONOR SHORTAGE

Over 81,000 patients are on the wait-list for transplantation in the United States today and more than 5000 will die this year without receiving a transplant. More startling is that almost 60% of those on the list today will die without receiving a transplant. Yet organs from deceased donors are recovered from less than 50% of actual, potential donors, resulting in the loss of thousands of life-saving transplants. Most of the small, annual 1-2% increase in the number of deceased donors has come from expanding the medical and social conditions previously used to eliminate potential donors, while the wait-list continues to grow at a rate of 12% annually.

UNOS CONSENT CONFERENCE

In late April, UNOS sponsored a national consensus conference, "Maximizing the Consent Process, From Research to Practice" in Orlando, Florida. Over 100 experts from the organ procurement and transplant community came together to address "best practices" for (1) training and maintaining recovery coordinators, (2) improving the consent process, (3) supporting the needs of the donor families, and (4) evaluating the impact of "first person consent" or "donor authorization". The recommendations from these work groups will soon be published and I will limit my discussion to those from the Work Group on "donor authorization" moderated by Helen Leslie, executive director of LifeNet OPO in Virginia and myself.

DONOR AUTHORIZATION

In 1968, the National Conference on Commissioners for Uniform State Laws drafted the Uniform Anatomical Gift Act (UAGA) that authorized anyone 18 years of age or more to "gift" any part of his body to take effect upon death and that this could not be rescinded without his consent by anyone. Over the next decade this was adopted by the legislatures of all 50 states. However, this was virtually ignored by all OPOs because of the small numbers of potential donors with legal donor documents and the difficulty in documenting their existence at the time of death. In 1995, the Center for Organ Recovery and Education (CORE), the OPO for western Pennsylvania and part of West Virginia, began accepting the donor document as legally binding. In the subsequent 7 years, they found that donation occurred 100% of the time when the donor document was available but only the usual 51% when consent from the family was utilized. The Work Group's recommendation was to develop an aggressive national effort to increase the recovery of donor organs by moving to an emphasis on the "donor authorization" process.

The Work Group then developed the following position:

1. The decedent's right to donate should take precedence in the donation process.
2. This should be accomplished in the framework of:
   a. honoring the donor's wishes
   b. respecting the needs of the recipient
   c. continuing to support and care for the donor family.
3. The approach should provide:
   a. a consistent level of support for the donor family
   b. sensitivity to the needs of diverse populations
   c. the achievement of an effective paradigm shift by hospital staff and donation specialists in the process for recovering organs.

An action agenda was developed to:

1. Create national synergy and momentum to:
   a. enlist a broad-based coalition within the procurement/transplant arena and government agencies
   b. seek allies from the general public and greater healthcare community
   c. explore the need for UAGA revisions
   d. advance a supportive public relations strategy
   e. pursue "donor rights" legislation in all 50 states
2. Promote donor registries as a vehicle for:
   a. a "national" donor card and depository
   b. "online", multiple access sites.

I am happy to report that in the short month following the conference, this proposal has been endorsed by the Executive Committee of the Association of Organ Procurement Organizations (AOPO), the Advisory Council on Organ Transplantation to the Secretary of Health and Human Services (ACOT), and is under discussion by the National Kidney Foundation, the Coalition on Donation, the American Society of Transplantation, and the American Society of Transplant Surgeons.

I am hopeful that over the next 2 years, this program could result in a significant increase in the number of our citizens willing to come forward and authorizing their "gift of life" to their fellow citizens in need.

Thank you.

Mr. GREENWOOD. Thank you Dr. Metzger.

The Chair recognizes himself for 10 minutes and I'd like to address my first question to Ms. Snyder.

HHS received the Advisory Committee on Transplantation's 18 recommendations in November. What has the Department done with the recommendations over the past 6 months since receiving them?

Ms. SNYDER. Over the last 6 months, a large part of that time has been spent understanding the recommendations, exploring those recommendations, making sure that all interested parties have been represented and have had an opportunity to bring those viewpoints to the table. There has been—as I'm sure you're aware, given the seriousness and the breadth of issues in the transplantation community, each one of the 18 recommendations has a great deal of follow-up work that we will need to do. Even though the Secretary has said that he agrees in principle to them, actually taking them and implementing and operationalizing them is now the point where we are, and now we plan to move forward.

The 18 recommendations were really divided into two groups, and the first 7 of them were really around ways to improve the safety of living donors. It was interesting that in 2001, I believe, the number of living donors for the first time exceeded the number of nonliving donors. And so that issue has become more and more pressing as to those rights and responsibilities around that set of individuals. And so many of the recommendations dealt with that and, for instance, informed consent standards to be implemented for all living donors. We've asked the OPTN to address those consent standards to make them available and to work them through, looking at, for instance, a data base of health outcomes for those people who are living donors, what happens to them after the process, and more in terms of longitudinal looks at their health.

And so the Secretary has asked NIH to look within their research protocols to accommodate that request so that they can see what is the best way to track outcomes and the best way to know what happens to that group of people to make sure that the living donation process is as safe as it can be and works as well as it can for that group of people.

Those are just some examples of the type of recommendations that came out of that committee.

There is also another group of them on ways to improve nonliving consent rates and the allocation process. What we've done is take each recommendation, say who is it that needs to work through it. The Secretary has formed work groups across the Department of Health and Human Services. The Centers for Medicare and Medicaid Services is certainly impacted by the recommendations, the National Institutes of Health is impacted by them, our partners in the private sector, the UNOS organization, certainly HRSA.

So now what we need to do is to take all of those and turn them, you know, into actual plans that can happen. And that's what we'll be doing.

Mr. GREENWOOD. Do you have a timeframe as to—anticipated timeframe that you anticipate that these recommendations will be in force?

Ms. SNYDER. I think it's different for each recommendation so I couldn't give you an average. Do we have a—so it's separate for each one. What we could do is provide the committee with our matrix of recommendations and our estimated timeframes.

Mr. GREENWOOD. Would you do that, please?

Ms. SNYDER. Certainly.

Mr. GREENWOOD. Do you have a sense of how long you think it will take before the targeted hospitals meet the goal of conversion rate of 75 percent?

Ms. SNYDER. That's an excellent question and, in fact, in preparing for this hearing it's one that I asked just yesterday. I think the answer to that is it's a little bit—if you will allow me, it's a little bit like losing weight. The first 20 pounds comes off pretty easily; the last 5 is really hard. So depending on the individual hospital and where it stands on that scale; is it someone who's already at 65 percent that you're trying to move to 75 percent; is it someone who is at 20 percent that you're trying to move to 50 percent? You know, which one is going to be harder? You know, getting it on this side of the scale.

We believe that the 75 percent is the target. I had hoped that we could be there within a year. The staff tells me that that would be a very, very ambitious goal, but that we do believe we will have significant increases in the 46 percent, but may not achieve the 75 percent in the first 12 to 18 months.

Mr. GREENWOOD. Have you calculated what the additional number of donors would be if you did get the hospitals to 75 percent?

Ms. SNYDER. I believe it was 6,000 organs a year would become available, which would be a significant increase.

Mr. GREENWOOD. That would—that's roughly equal to the shortage, is it not?

Ms. SNYDER. That's correct.

Mr. GREENWOOD. Okay.

Dr. Metzger, you discussed the fact that OPOs have difficulty documenting a decedent's intent to donate at the time of death. Yet for donor authorization to be effective, documentation of the decedent's intent is critical. So how do you propose that this be done?

Mr. METZGER. Well, this has always been a difficult problem in the country and there's always been a lot of naysayers. And to me it seems like with modern technology that we should be able to overcome this. We have smart cards now that people can carry around with them with their medical history and different things. We have computer technology, where there are, I heard on CNN last—2 months ago—there are 750 million active MasterCard and Visa cards in the United States. We're dealing with looking at signing up 150 or 200 million people. And with the ability with modern technology, I think we can create registries that we will have access to onsite in the hospital with modern technology.

Mr. GREENWOOD. What is the status of registries?

Mr. METZGER. Registries, I think, are mired in remote technology. They often have 386 computers, the inability to input data. But they're becoming more effective. We are actually using ours daily in the State of Florida now. We have scanned in documents of wills.

Mr. GREENWOOD. It's done on a State-by-State basis.

Mr. METZGER. Yes.

Mr. GREENWOOD. And how many States have registries, do you know?

Mr. METZGER. I'm not sure the exact number, but it's a little over a majority now, I think.

Mr. GREENWOOD. Is there a reason to have one central Federal registry?

Mr. METZGER. I think this would be an optimal way to do it. But there already are State registries that are operational, and it might be easier to make them transparent across State lines and utilize that mechanism rather than——

Mr. GREENWOOD. You said there are naysayers. What are the arguments?

Mr. METZGER. The argument was that you have to enroll several—or many millions of people to get to the 15,000 to 20,000 potential donors out there in any 1 year. But I think that's possible today.

Mr. GREENWOOD. Are there confidentiality issues that make this difficult?

Mr. METZGER. I don't think so. The people that work in this area tell me that you can have very secure networks. In fact, one of the concerns of OPOs has always been how would they know that the potential donor hasn't rescinded his documentation?

Mr. GREENWOOD. Right.

Mr. METZGER. And that's always a problem with that with donor cards. But if we had this on line with an access site, all they have to do is call 1-800 and say for some reason, no, I don't want to do it anymore, and it's there. So it has opportunities on both ends.

Mr. GREENWOOD. And are there those who argue that names might get on registries that don't belong on registries?

Mr. METZGER. Well, there's always the potential of that, but there are secure ways of making these registries.

Mr. GREENWOOD. Okay. Later this morning we will be hearing from the AMA about the policies it adopted last summer recommending studies of the impact of financial incentives on donations. Has UNOS addressed this issue; and, if so, how?

Mr. METZGER. Yes. UNOS, a year and a half ago, endorsed the proposal to look at studies and support the study of financial incentives to see if there would be any benefit in the organ donation process with financial incentives. In essence it backed the AMA stance.

Mr. GREENWOOD. In order to study the impact of financial incentives, you actually have to provide them, don't you. It's pretty hard to study it hypothetically?

Mr. METZGER. Yes. You would need actual data.

Mr. GREENWOOD. So we would have to actually in some pilot way offer financial incentives to see what the response rate is and see if that differs from some other group. Does HRSA or HHS have a stated position with regard to financial incentives?

Ms. SNYDER. I think the position has been—very much played out in the discussion among yourselves this morning that there are many different points of view, and those points of view need to be fully examined before moving forward with a public policy. I do know that the ACOT has agreed that this year it will take up the issue of financial incentives, and we are looking very much forward to the results of those deliberations and discussions because there is a great representation of the community and those impacted in the community within that group.

Mr. GREENWOOD. My time has expired. The gentlelady from Colorado is recognized for 10 minutes.

Ms. DeGETTE. Dr. Metzger, I don't want to put words in your mouth but what I am hearing you and others say is part of the problem we have is that hospitals don't have accurate information as to whether someone has made the decision to donate their organs or not, correct?

Mr. METZGER. Correct.

Ms. DeGETTE. And so one thing we're trying to figure out, and I agree completely with this, is how to improve our registries. So that if I go down to the driver's license bureau, or however else I do it, and say, "Yes, I want to be an organ donor," when I am lying there brain dead on life support there's some way that the medical personnel will know that, irrespective of whether my family has provided that information or not, right?

Mr. METZGER. Right.

Ms. DeGETTE. And Ms. Snyder, it sounds to me like your targets are to try to get it up to 75 percent at the 200 hospitals where they are doing most of the donations; is that right?

Ms. SNYDER. That's correct.

Ms. DeGETTE. And certainly, registries would help with that, because health care personnel would then know did someone agree or not and they wouldn't have to rely on distraught family members or incomplete information, right?

Ms. SNYDER. I think our issue from HHS's perspective is that it is a matter of State law, which is what governs the establishment of those kinds of registries where people consent and who can revoke it and who can honor the wishes of those individuals who have given consent. The approach we have been looking at is taking model legislation, if you will, to try to get States to at first address the issue of making sure you have a nonrevokable agreement to donate and then moving from that point to the registry.

Ms. DEGETTE. Right. And if you had that, it would make the decisions a lot more clear, right?

Ms. SNYDER. It would make the decisions more clear. I think the issue around registries is one that people don't like to talk about, but it is simply the technology is probably there, but it becomes the issue of funding for it, who would maintain the registries, how would you ensure that privacy rights are protected.

Ms. DEGETTE. I don't want to interrupt you, but you are exactly right. But what the Federal Government has done with other kinds of registries, sex offender registries, we put resources into them— you know, DWAI registries. We put resources into helping States to coordinate and update their registries, and this is something we can easily do with organ donation registries. Do you think that would be a financial need that you would see down the road?

Ms. SNYDER. There would definitely be a cost of establishing any kind of data base that would interface.

Ms. DEGETTE. What just occurred to me, while I was listening to Dr. Metzger, Mr. Chairman, is that this idea that the chairman has of giving financial incentives to donors to agree to donate, that may not be the thing that solves this problem. You could say to me, okay, I am going to give you a $10,000 life insurance policy if you agree to donate your organs. But if I am hit in a car crash, and I am in a hospital and no one knows about that, it doesn't matter. It sounds to me like, if we worked on the issue of donor registration and education, that that might go a long way to solving the problem.

What do you think about that, Dr. Metzger?

Mr. METZGER. We do have to adopt the donor registration process prior to the next step, whichever that might be. Once we do that, we have to figure out how to get people to sign the card and sign on.

Ms. DEGETTE. Sounds like a lot of people are signing up, and we could always use more. Don't get me wrong. I think there are a lot of things we can do to get people to agree to be donors. But it seems to me that just today, today, if you could have hospitals, particularly these top 200 hospitals, knowing that someone had agreed to be a donor, and if you had an irrevocable donation decision that was there, that would help a lot more in the short-term with getting more organs.

Mr. METZGER. It's definitely a need. And it would take a significant segment of that population where you only have 51 percent consenting into that population where you have 100 percent donation.

Ms. DeGette. Right. Ms. Snyder, before when I was asking Mr. Roth the question about what kinds of public service announcements, and so on, that have been made, you were nodding. I wonder if you could expand to the answer to that question.

Ms. Snyder. As part of the Secretary's initiative to increase donation rates, there have been a number of education activities that have been launched and are being launched. One component of that includes some dollars from the increased appropriation that we received for this activity that will go to radio and television ad campaigns in the 15 biggest markets. So there is a small dollar amount.

Ms. DeGette. How much is it?

Ms. Snyder. I think it is about $1 million. And a number of public service announcements would supplement that, in addition to what we would have to pay to do the ads.

The other thing that I think is really exciting around the education efforts are two initiatives that I think are very important. One is a workplace partnership. The Secretary had a goal of signing up 5,000 businesses by April 2003, and to date, we have actually enrolled over 7200 businesses. And part of that is just having the, if you will, the poster at the watercooler that says "have you thought about donation?" and making it something that's on peoples' minds.

Another part that we're doing around education is school-based education curricula, where we're hitting the group from age 10 to 22 through various educational interventions. And one to me that anybody who has teenage children knows that the first place that kids pay attention is drivers' ed. So introducing it in drivers' ed, I think, will start the conversation. That is more a long-term strategy. You have got to start the education campaign and that is a long-term strategy, and get people when they're young to start to think about it.

Ms. DeGette. Have there been any studies done to show the effect of public education on increasing organ donation rates?

Ms. Snyder. I don't know that it has been specific to organ donation rates, but certainly folks have looked at what happened around seat belt laws, what happened around helmet laws.

Ms. DeGette. Do you think that would be an interesting study to see if increased public service announcements work—otherwise, why make the effort if it is not making a difference?

Ms. Snyder. I think it would be interesting, but I think this is one of those where you can look at research that has already been done in the community, and perhaps rather than putting funds forward to do that, you can extrapolate to it.

Ms. DeGette. Dr. Metzger, are you aware of any efforts that the donation networks have made? I go back to this diabetes example where some of the private diabetes organizations have really worked with religious leaders and others to educate.

Mr. Metzger. Over the past 20 years, we spent millions of dollars in public education but haven't gotten too far with it, and one of your comments was about some of the public ads that are usually on at 3 o'clock in the morning. We actually had—one of our recovery coordinators thought during one of the shuttle launches, why don't we have astronauts sign organ donor cards in space, and she got NASA to do it. Unfortunately, they wouldn't tell us when the signing was going to be. It was 2:30 one morning when they found time to do it. So there weren't very many people watching it. It's hard to get the public education.

We have a very successful program called Get Carded at universities in Florida. We started it in Orlando at the University of Central Florida. We distributed over 85,000 donor cards to college students. And we know in looking at it that 80 percent of them sign on to the card. We expanded that into the University of Florida, University of South Florida and Florida Atlantic University. So these are some things that you have to get really almost one to one with these people to get them to think about this. Billboards, TV ads and that, when you are not even thinking about dying and donations, don't make that big of an impact.

Ms. DeGETTE. That's why I'm thinking of efforts with the churches, this effort that Mr. Roth was talking about to get the ministers preaching from the pulpit, but then to have people there with the cards to get people to sign up.

Mr. METZGER. All of our OPOs have programs to do that. And then you have to look at the demographics. In the African American community, usually my generation of African Americans respond very positively to the clergy. When you go down to the next generation, it may be sports figures and community leaders. So you have to get to all those groups.

I would like to say one thing about the OPTN and pediatrics, if I may. We have established preferential allocation to children. In the kidney program, children under the age of 11 get four extra points in the allocation process. And over the age of 11 to 18, they get three extra points and they carry those past age 18. For a lot of the other organs, the problem is the size. You can't put big adult organs in children. So they need child organs, but you can put segments of adult organs into children. So there has been, over the last 5 years, considerable movement to using liver segments and lung segments in children for transplantation.

Unfortunately, the heart has to be the size of the individual, but there are very few pediatric hearts, if any, going to adults because they don't size. Pediatric——

Ms. DeGETTE. Do they give extra points for the heart?

Mr. METZGER. The heart and liver programs are primarily based on a severity of illness process now, but there is a separate one for children.

Ms. DeGETTE. Thank you.

Mr. GREENWOOD. The Chair thanks the gentlelady.

The gentleman from Oregon is recognized for 10 minutes.

Mr. WALDEN. Thank you, Mr. Chairman.

We talked about public service announcements. I wonder if your agencies are looking into what the National Guard bureaus are doing around the State with what's called an NCSA, noncommercial spot announcement where they work with broadcast associations in each State, make a donation to the State in return for multiples of announcements that run. As a broadcaster, I am somewhat familiar with the program, and it has worked very effectively.

Ms. SNYDER. I am not aware of any efforts, but we will take that suggestion back, and we're certainly looking for ways to get the word out and do it in the most cost effective way we can.

Mr. WALDEN. Sometimes it as much as 7 or 8 to 1. The stations donate the time, and the moneys go to the State associations, and I think for many organizations, it has been very helpful. I know the situation in the Oregon Health Plan, the State got involved in trying to get employers involved in some things, and based on marked increase in participation after the in NCSA campaign ran it, it might be a way to stretch your million dollars nationwide. And I congratulate you on signing up those 7,200 businesses. And I think it will enure to the benefit of the program. Mr. Chairman, I really have no questions from this distinguished panel, and I appreciate your input and your work, and I yield back my time.

Mr. GREENWOOD. The Chair thanks the gentleman.

And the Chair thanks our witnesses and we excuse you now.

And for everyone's information, we will have a series of votes probably in about half an hour, but I would like to call the next panel forward and at least take their testimony before we have to break for votes, and maybe have to return after votes for questions.

We would invite Tim Olsen, Community Development Coordinator for the Wisconsin Donor Network; Mr. Robert Sade, M.D., Professor of Surgery at the Medical University of South Carolina; Mr. Richard DeVos from Michigan; Dr. Joseph Vacanti, M.D., Director of Pediatric Transplantation, Massachusetts General Hospital; Dr. Abraham Shaked, M.D., President of the American Society of Transplant Surgeons; and Dr. Francis L. Delmonico, M.D., of the National Kidney Foundation. Welcome all of you. Thank you for your patience. I think all of you have been present. As I informed the previous panels and that this is an investigative hearing, and it is our practice to take testimony for these hearings under oath, and I ask if you object to giving your testimony under oath. Okay. I need to advise you pursuant to the rules of this committee and the House, you are entitled to be represented by counsel. Any of you wish to be represented counsel? The Enron folks did, but most others don't.

I would ask if you would stand and raise your right hands, please.

[Witnesses sworn.]

Mr. GREENWOOD. I believe we will begin with Mr. Olsen.

TESTIMONY OF TIM OLSEN, COMMUNITY DEVELOPMENT CO-ORDINATOR, WISCONSIN DONOR NETWORK; ROBERT M. SADE, PROFESSOR OF SURGERY, MEDICAL UNIVERSITY OF SOUTH CAROLINA; RICHARD M. DEVOS; JOSEPH P. VACANTI, DIRECTOR OF PEDIATRIC TRANSPLANTATION, MASSACHU-SETTS GENERAL HOSPITAL; ABRAHAM SHAKED, PRESIDENT, AMERICAN SOCIETY OF TRANSPLANT SURGEONS; AND FRANCIS L. DELMONICO, NATIONAL KIDNEY FOUNDATION

Mr. OLSEN. Thank you very much for inviting the Wisconsin Donor Network to be represented at this hearing. It's an honor for us to participate, and we applaud your efforts to increase organ donation.

Wisconsin Donor Network is one of two organ procurement organizations in Wisconsin. There are also three tissue banks and an eye bank. We all work together in many ways, but also pursue awareness opportunities as individual organizations and have each been very successful with our organ and tissue recovery efforts. With that in mind, I am only speaking on behalf of the Wisconsin Donor Network today, not all of the State organizations.

Wisconsin is often looked to as an excellent donor State, and we are very proud of that status. Unfortunately, we have no way of knowing what we have done, if anything, that has made donation in Wisconsin so successful. We don't have a registry, and we don't have any methods of determining how many people act on our awareness efforts. I can share with you many characteristics and programs that we believe have made a positive impact on donation in Wisconsin.

Two of the biggest influencing factors over the past 10 to 15 years, I believe, are our former Governor and our successful transplant center. During Tommy Thompson's 14 years as Wisconsin Governor, he was the State's biggest proponent of organ donation. He was very outspoken about it, as he continues to be, and serves as an excellent leader for organ donation awareness throughout Wisconsin. He also implemented an annual ceremony and Governor's Medal to honor donors and their families, a tradition we expect to continue this summer, its tenth year.

We have also benefited from having four outstanding transplant centers in the State. Even though Wisconsin is only the 18th most populated State, only seven other States in the country performed more transplants than the 796 that took place in Wisconsin last year.

One successful transplant center is returning their patients to their homes, jobs, schools, churches and social circles. That shows others, by example, that organ donation is saving lives and a great way to help others which, in turn, makes others inclined to donate.

We have also tried to be aggressive with our awareness activities. Wisconsin Donor Network relies on the assistance of 300 outstanding volunteers, almost all of whom have a personal connection to donation as transplant recipients, family members of recipients or family members of donors. They speak to groups about their experience, hand out information and answer questions at health fairs and special events and serve as great examples of the success and importance of organ donation and transplant.

We also staff the Wisconsin Donor Network information booth at the Wisconsin State Fair and other county fairs. Last year more than 1,100 people signed up to be donors at our three fair booths, and nearly 2,500 people took donor information or materials at the booths.

We hold an annual run/walk, Sarah's Stride, held in memory of a local teenager who died while awaiting a transplant. The fifth annual Sarah's Stride 3 weeks ago attracted more than 1,250 participants and raised more than $55,000 for donor awareness efforts in Wisconsin. The funds raised through Sarah's Stride and other donations are used to fund special donor awareness projects.

One of the most important projects that it funded, and continues to fund, is the drivers' education curriculum that we developed to provide to drivers' education instructors. In the summer of 2000, Wisconsin passed a law requiring at least 30 minutes of organ and tissue donation information as part of drivers' education programs. To support that mandate, the Wisconsin Donor Network developed a curriculum tailored for drivers' education instructors to use in the classroom and provided it at no cost to every drivers' education program in the State that fall. A few months later, in early 2001, the Wisconsin Donor Network finished a more comprehensive curriculum on organ and tissue donation for health education instructors and sent it free to every high school in the State.

We are very proud of our Wisconsin Coalition on Donation, which is a group of organizations with a common interest in donation from throughout the State that have joined together to work on awareness project that we ordinarily wouldn't be able to address at the State level on our own. Both State organ procurement organizations, all three tissue banks, the eye bank, a blood bank, the kidney liver and heart associations and others have spearheaded some very successful awareness efforts in the past 2 years and continues to increase its efforts.

More recently the Wisconsin Donor Network launched its Website, which is a little more than a year old. Traffic to the Website continues to grow and serves as a great online resource for organ donation information for State residents.

Also last year, the Wisconsin Donor Network developed its own television ad and for the first time, committed to a substantial paid advertising campaign. We chose to target women in our service area, aged 35 to 54, for several reasons, and ran the ad throughout 2002. We have no way of knowing what effect, if any, the ad had, but we do know that our 2002 consent rate of 66 percent was significantly higher than the national average, which is typically measured at between 45 and 54 percent. Even more dramatic, our donations increased 33 percent from 2001 to 2002. That 33 percent increase contrasts with the 1.6 percent overall national increase last year and was the third highest increase of all organ procurement organizations in the Nation last year.

Thank you for allowing me to provide a brief overview of our efforts in Wisconsin. We truly appreciate your interest in this very important public issue.

[The prepared statement of Tim Olsen follows:]

PREPARED STATEMENT OF TIM OLSEN, COMMUNITY DEVELOPMENT COORDINATOR, WISCONSIN DONOR NETWORK

Thank you very much for inviting the Wisconsin Donor Network to be represented at this hearing. It's an honor for us to participate and we applaud your efforts to increase organ donation.

The Wisconsin Donor Network is one of two organ procurement organizations in Wisconsin. There are also three tissue banks and an eye bank. We all work together in many ways, but also pursue awareness opportunities as individual organizations and have each been very successful with our organ and tissue recovery efforts. With that in mind, I am only speaking on behalf of the Wisconsin Donor Network today, not all of these state organizations.

Wisconsin is often looked to as an excellent donor state and we're very proud of that status. Unfortunately, we have no way of knowing what we have done, if anything, that has made donation in Wisconsin so successful. We don't have a registry and we don't have any methods of determining how many people act on our awareness efforts. I can, though, share with you many characteristics and programs that we believe have made a positive impact on donation in Wisconsin.

Two of the biggest influencing factors over the past 10-15 years, I believe, are our former governor and our successful transplant centers. During Tommy Thompson's 14 years as Wisconsin governor, he was the state's biggest proponent of organ donation. We was very outspoken about it, as he continues to be, and served as an excellent leader for organ donation awareness throughout Wisconsin. He also implemented an annual ceremony and governor's medal to honor donors and their families, a tradition that we expect to continue this summer, its 10th year.

We have also benefited from having four outstanding transplant centers in the state. Even though Wisconsin is only the 18th most populated state, only seven other states in the country performed more transplants than the 796 that took place in Wisconsin last year. When successful transplant centers are returning their patients to their homes, jobs, schools, churches and social circles, that shows others by example that organ donation is saving lives and is a great way to help others, which in turn makes others more inclined to donate.

We have also tried to be aggressive with our awareness activities. The Wisconsin Donor Network relies on the assistance of 300 outstanding volunteers, almost all of whom have a personal connection to donation as transplant recipients, family members of recipients, or family members of donors. They speak to groups about their experience, hand out information and answer questions at health fairs and special events and just serve as great examples of the success and importance of donation and transplant.

They also staff the Wisconsin Donor Network information booths at the Wisconsin State Fair and other county fairs. Last year more than 1,100 people signed up to be donors at our three fair booths, and nearly 2,500 people took donor information or materials at the booths.We hold an annual run/walk, Sarah's Stride, held in honor and memory of a local teenager who died while awaiting a transplant. The fifth annual Sarah's Stride three weeks ago attracted more than 1,250 participants and raised more than $55,000 for donor awareness efforts in Wisconsin.

The funds raised through Sarah's Stride and other donations are used to fund special donor awareness projects. One of the most important projects that it funded, and continues to fund, is the driver's education curriculum that we developed to provide to drivers' education instructors. In the summer of 2000 Wisconsin passed a law requiring at least 30 minutes of organ and tissue donation information as part of drivers' education programs. To support that mandate, the Wisconsin Donor Network developed a curriculum tailored for driver's education instructors to use in the classroom and provided it at no cost to every drivers' education program in the state that fall. A few months later, in early 2001, the Wisconsin Donor Network finished a more comprehensive curriculum on organ and tissue donation for health education instructors and sent it free to every high school in the state.

We're also very proud of our Wisconsin Coalition on Donation, which is a group of organizations with a common interest in donation from throughout the state that have joined together to work on awareness projects that we ordinarily wouldn't be able to address at the state level on our own. Both state organ procurement organizations, all three tissue banks, the eye bank, a blood bank, the kidney, liver, lung and heart associations, and others have spearheaded some very successful awareness events within the past two years and continues to increase its efforts.

More recently, the Wisconsin Donor Network launched its website, which is now a little more than a year old. Traffic to the website continues to grow as it serves as a great on-line resource for organ donation information for state residents.

Also last year, the Wisconsin Donor Network developed its own television ad and for the first time committed to a substantial paid advertising campaign. We chose to target women in our service area, age 35 to 54, for several reasons, and ran the ad throughout 2002. We have no way of knowing what effect, if any, the ad had, but we do know that our 2002 consent rate of 66 percent was significantly higher than the national average, which is typically measured at between 45 and 54 percent. Even more dramatic, our donations increased 33 percent from 2001 to 2002. That 33 percent increase contrasts with the 1.6 percent overall national increase last year and was the third highest increase of all organ procurement organizations in the nation last year. (VHS tape of the ad available.)

Thank you for allowing me provide a brief overview of our efforts in Wisconsin. We truly appreciate your interest in this very important public health issue.

Mr. GREENWOOD. Thank you Mr. Olsen.

Dr. Sade.

TESTIMONY OF ROBERT M. SADE

Mr. SADE. Good afternoon, and thank you, Chairman Greenwood, for inviting the American Medical Association to participate in today's hearing. In particular, Mr. Chairman, we thank you for your leadership in this particular issue which we take as very important.

I am Dr. Robert Sade, a member of the AMA's Council on Ethical and Judicial Affairs. I'm a cardiothoracic surgeon and Medical Director of the Organ Procurement Organization for South Carolina. AMA policy is developed through a broadly representative process involving physician delegates from every State, over 100 national medical specialty societies, Federal service agencies and other groups. You have heard already about the 6,000 deaths a year while organs are not being donated but rather are buried or cremated, so I won't pursue that any further.

AMA policy developed last year supports the scientific study of financial incentives and other motivators to increase the supply of organ donations from patients who recently died. This policy was recommended by the AMA Ethics Council on the grounds that financial incentives are not intrinsically unethical, but may be ethical depending upon the balance of benefits and harms as established by factual data. Currently, there is no scientific data showing whether modest financial incentives, such as direct payments to families, tax credits, funeral reimbursements, or charitable contributions would increase or decrease the supply of organs.

Almost all of the arguments against financial incentives are based on assumptions that could be proven or disproven by scientifically designed studies. Factual evidence could determine the presence or absence of harm to individuals, groups or society as a whole and resolve many of the policy debates about financial incentives. Therefore, the AMA supports studying the impact of moderate financial incentives and other motivators on cadaveric organ donation.

I would like to make two important points. First, the studies should apply only to organ donation. The current system of organ distribution should be continued under UNOS guidelines. In other words, no one could buy an organ. Second, studies should be limited to understanding motivation only for donation from newly deceased patients and not for donation by living donors. Scientific design is essential, so each study should be limited to a small, but broadly representative population segment, should provide financial incentives at the lowest level that could reasonably be expected to increase organ donation, should have measurable outcomes to assess their effectiveness and should be completed within defined timeframes.

The studies should not only measure the effect of incentives on donation rates but also on the public perception of the meaning of organ donation. Studies should be undertaken only after three things occur. First, a new law would be needed for the purpose of collecting data on financial incentives. Currently the National Organ Transplantation Act prohibits providing any valuable consideration for organ donation. Second, guidance and advice should be sought from the particular under study to assure that the proposed research is consistent with their needs, values and mores.

And third, protocols that meet ethical standards and are scientifically rigorous must be reviewed and approved by appropriate oversight bodies, such as institutional review boards. All ethical safeguards that generally guide the participation of human subjects and clinical research should be followed when studying the impact of financial incentives on organ donation rates.

Last year, Chairman Greenwood introduced legislation that would have authorized the Department of Health and Human Services to carry out demonstration projects to increase the supply of organs donated for human transplantation. Such demonstration projects, if scientifically designed, would be an important first step in exploring the motivation behind cadaveric organ donation.

Once again Mr. Chairman, thank you for inviting us to testify before you today.

[The prepared statement of Robert M. Sade follows:]

PREPARED STATEMENT OF ROBERT M. SADE ON BEHALF OF THE AMERICAN MEDICAL ASSOCIATION

The American Medical Association (AMA) appreciates the opportunity to share its views on appropriate strategies to increase organ donation rates and thanks Chairman Greenwood and members of the Subcommittee for holding today's hearing on this important issue.

BACKGROUND

In the United States, there is a striking gap between the demand for transplantable organs and the available supply of such organs. Annually, approximately 6,000 patients with end-stage organ failure—the equivalent of 16 per day—die because of the lack of available organs. Successes of solid-organ transplantation have greatly increased the need for organ donors. Unfortunately, donation rates have not kept up with the need for organs which has grown nearly five times faster than the number of cadaveric donors. The annually compounded rate (1990-2000) of increase in number of patients on waiting lists has averaged 14.1% a year. Meanwhile, the rate of increase of donors has averaged only 2.9% a year. Unrealized potential accounts for much of the donation gap, with studies suggesting that each year only 35-50% of potential donors consent to donation. Because the number of potential donors far exceeds current procurement rates, the AMA, like many other groups, has identified the urgent need to develop new strategies to increase donation rates in an effort to alleviate our country's organ shortage.

THE NEED FOR INNOVATIVE APPROACHES

In the past, initiatives to increase organ donation have included vigorous educational campaigns to motivate individuals to become donors. Other efforts have been directed at health professionals urging them to educate patients regarding donation, or legislatively mandating that they present relatives of a newly deceased with a choice to donate. All these initiatives have been expanded through the establishment of the Organ Procurement and Transplantation Network (OPTN), donor card programs and donor registries, and the creation of specialized organ donation teams within hospitals that discuss organ donation with patients and families. Unfortunately, these efforts have failed to increase cadaveric donation rates significantly.

The AMA believes that these efforts should be maintained. It is essential that physicians and other organ donation advocates continue to promote voluntary donation of organs. Beyond these programs, however, the AMA supports innovative approaches that are informed by a more comprehensive understanding of what motivates and what hinders individuals' decisions to donate.

REEXAMINING DONOR MOTIVATION

The AMA applauds recent efforts by various groups to determine best practices in organ donation. Thorough study of these practices and their replication should increase donation rates.

The AMA applauds the attention that has been given to the issue of organ donation by the Secretary of Health and Human Services, Tommy Thompson. Under his leadership, the membership of the Advisory Committee on Organ Transplantation (ACOT) has doubled in size, and, it has successfully pursued its mission to enhance organ donation by ensuring that the system of organ transplantation is grounded in the best available medical science, while assuring the public that the system is as effective and equitable as possible. In November 2002, the ACOT issued a set of recommendations to the Secretary, some pertaining to the effectiveness of living donation and appropriate protection of potential living donors, and others relating to increasing the supply of organs from deceased donors.

Similarly, the United Network for Organ Sharing (UNOS) convened organ donation and transplantation professionals last month to build a consensus on best practices regarding techniques related to donation requests. Considering that the most common reason for missed donation opportunities is denial by the donor's family, this conference marked a concerted national effort to improve consent rates by examining shared characteristics among professionals who are routinely successful when approaching families and potential donors about organ donation. These findings, once implemented, could lead to increased rates of donation.

Creative proposals must continue to be examined for their potential to increase the number of cadaveric donations to help supplement current initiatives and address the shortage. Whether expanding criteria for donation, systematizing the use of asystolic donors, or incorporating organ donation as a specialized form of end-of-life care, ethical strategies should be investigated to establish their effectiveness in raising donation rates.

Against this background, the AMA recently considered issues related to donor motivation. We acknowledged the medical profession's obligation to continue to encourage the voluntary donation of organs in appropriate circumstances and also to support innovative approaches. We have noted that financial incentives might be an important motivational factor in the context of cadaveric organ donation but that it remains inadequately explored because of federal prohibition. In our view, such incentives are not intrinsically unethical even though they are counter to current customs, and, if proven effective, could save the lives of many patients suffering from end-stage organ failure.

ENCOURAGING THE STUDY OF FINANCIAL INCENTIVES

In June 2002, the AMA adopted a policy encouraging the medical community to support the reexamination of motivation for cadaveric organ donation. In particular, the report explored financial incentives as a possible strategy to increase organ donation, and recommended that the impact of these incentives on donation rates be studied. Theoretical concerns regarding harms that could result from offering financial incentives for organ donation were carefully considered:

- Currently, individuals see donation as a gift. To put a financial incentive on cadaveric organ donation might deter some individuals from wanting to be donors.
- Financial incentives for cadaveric organ donation might fuel what is considered by some as a disturbing trend towards viewing the human body as a source of profit.
- Payments might be unduly coercive to certain segments of the population, interfering with the voluntary nature of donation.
- Even if financial incentives initially are permitted for cadaveric organ donation only, pressure might build to allow payments to live donors.

Several of these concerns led a panel of experts convened by the American Society of Transplant Surgeons (ASTS), in April 2002, to oppose any form of direct payment for cadaveric organs. The panel was asked to determine whether an ethically acceptable pilot trial could be designed whereby a family would be offered a financial incentive to consent to the donation of organs from a deceased relative. The panel unanimously agreed that such direct payment would violate the standard of altruism in organ donation, leading to a system that would commodify human organs. The panel was divided with regard to the acceptability of other indirect incentives such as funeral reimbursements or charitable contributions, which would convey society's appreciation to a family for their gift of life.

For its part, the AMA notes that there is a dearth of scientific data supporting those concerns. Nearly all of the arguments against financial incentives are based on assumptions that can be proven or disproved by objective empirical studies. Factual evidence that would determine the presence or absence of harm to individuals, groups of individuals, or society as a whole could resolve many of the policy debates between those who object to financial incentives for cadaveric organ donation and those who favor such incentives. It is on this basis that the AMA supports the study of motivation, to gain a better understanding of the impact of moderate financial incentives and other motivators on cadaveric organ donation. Whether or not such incentives and other motivators are ethical depends, at least in part, upon the balance of benefits and harms that result from them.

In its June 2002 policy, the AMA articulated parameters for research studies investigating the effects of financial incentives for cadaveric organ donation. First and foremost, these studies should apply only to organ donation; the current system of organ distribution, as developed and administered by the United Network for Organ Sharing should be maintained. Also, the studies should be limited to understanding motivation for cadaveric organ donation only, and not its effect on living donors.

With respect to their design, each study should be limited to a small population, provide financial incentives at the lowest level that could reasonably be expected to increase organ donation, have measurable outcome variables to assess their effectiveness, and be completed within defined time frames. Altogether, it would be desirable that data be gathered from broad population segments and that they not only help measure the effect of incentives upon donation rates but also on public perception of the transplant enterprise and of the meaning of organ donation.

Moreover, studies should be undertaken only after:

- A new law is enacted for the purpose of collecting these data which would waive the National Organ Transplantation Act's legal prohibition against providing valuable considerations for organ donation.
- Guidance and advice have been sought from the particular population under study to ensure that the proposed research is consistent with their needs, values, and mores.
- Protocols that meet ethical standards and are scientifically rigorous have been reviewed and approved by appropriate oversight bodies, such as Institutional Review Boards.

All other ethical safeguards that generally guide the participation of human subjects in clinical investigations also should be adhered to when studying the impact of financial incentives on organ donation rates.

Models have been proposed by several organizations, including the ASTS and UNOS, whose Board of Directors agreed, days after the AMA adopted its policy, to support legislation that would enable studying the impact of incentives to encourage organ donation and to honor organ donors. Among the suggested models are: future contracts, as was proposed in a bill before Congress several years ago, that would have allowed for the implementation of a tax credit of up to $10,000 on the estate of the deceased donor; reimbursement for funeral expenses, as was passed into law in Pennsylvania, but was never implemented because of the federal prohibition; charitable donations; direct payment; and medals of honor. Moreover, Congressman Greenwood's leadership with this issue was displayed through the introduction of H.R. 5224 during the last Congress which would have authorized the Department of Health and Human Services to carry out demonstration projects to increase the supply of organs donated for human transplantation.

The potential benefits to be gained from each proposal discussed above remain speculative and must be weighed against possible harms before any such program is widely implemented. For example, if research shows that little discernable harm to potential donors, their families, or society results from offering modest financial incentives, thereby saving more lives through increased organ donation rate, everyone benefits. But if serious harms are found, physicians and policymakers will need to search for other means of increasing donation rates.

A thorough discussion of this matter also must include consideration of the costs of foregoing such studies. Currently patients die each day waiting for available organs. Therefore, a better informed debate is necessary, one that can occur only after the effectiveness of various incentive models has been measured. It is for this reason that the AMA will continue to advocate for the study of financial incentives as a strategy for increasing organ donation.

We thank the members of the Subcommittee for initiating a review of this important matter and for inviting the AMA to share its views.

Mr. GREENWOOD. Thank you very much.

Mr. DeVos.

TESTIMONY OF RICHARD M. DEVOS

Mr. DeVos. Sounds like I am the lightning rod. I am the only person here not a doctor or not involved in this organization or industry. I am just a heart recipient, 6 years and 1 month ago today

I received my new life. I was 71 years old at the time. I am now 77. My heart is now 45, so my average age is 60.

Anyway, I thank God for the miracle that brought me a new heart. Therefore, I have no interest in this, other than a citizen trying to get involved and do something in gratefulness for my new heart. I began to wonder what we could do and why this line was flat on finding new organs. So I engaged my first heart physician, who did my first bypass surgery to work for me full-time to try to find out what we could do to make a difference in getting more organs so other people can be blessed. So I am grateful to you, Chairman Greenwood, for your interest and inquiry. And I am just a citizen trying to make a difference in this whole process.

Being a business guy, I kind of come down to, if you want more of something, pay for it. I understand all the rest of it and all the promotion and all the effort we ought to go into to give it PR and give it effort, but why don't you give the money to the person who gives the organ and maybe we will get some further organ donation. So I come down on that side and we tried to fashion a way to do this. I am way off what I propose doing here. But first of all, we support making the donor the real person who signs that card, make that stick and make it count. And I don't care how you work the donor lists. You'll get it all done, and I think we'll have a huge impact.

Now, once we do that, we go on to say how do we get people to sign the card, and how do we increase the number of people who will sign the card, and especially for the young people who we are seeking the most to do this. And so we thought throw some money at it. Now, I know that is not very sophisticated, but I say let's test it and find out. And so we said, throw $10,000 on the table and see how many people will jump and say I'll sign for that. And when we look at that in the realm of talking of $6,000 or $7,000 at— 7,000 organs at $10,000, it doesn't amount to much, not compared to the savings that will exist by getting people off dialysis and getting them some life and hope for their future.

And so we come down to the simple conclusion, let's see what we can do. Give us a chance to do a little financial test and see if we can excite a whole bunch of people.

Now, this is not our idea. It was originally proposed by somebody in Greenwood's district. Project Donor was done by Gene Epstein and Al Boessmann, and they were the first ones who brought it to our attention. So we got on board with them and said let's see if we can can't get somewhere with this. We are carrying the mail for them. We decided that it was worthy of a test. And I couldn't believe the resistance I ran into when I tried to do this. It was just kind of a wow, what is wrong? I kind of felt like the people who write about this are not on the waiting list like I was. If you're on the waiting list, you'll have a different view on this whole subject whether or not it's okay to throw a little money at somebody. So I know we will need to have sign up millions of people, but that's what we need. We need millions of people to sign up, so we can get down to that 6 or 7 or 10,000 people that will do it. They're there, they're available, and if we launch that campaign, put the money in the hands of the people who will sign the cards, and maybe we'll get somewhere, but at least find out.

I salute Tommy Thompson for all his efforts. We had a wonderful visit with him up at that Department and talked about all of this. We're concerned with the minorities who are fearful of things of this type. But if you put them on the list and keep it confidential, and it's not available until someone is brain dead, then you check the list, then nobody has to be fearful of all of this. This is not something to be afraid of. I know the joy of it. I met my donor and my donor was so happy to talk to me and be grateful. She came out of the room 1 day and said, "Did you get a heart on June 2?" and I said, "Yes." she said, "You have my heart." Fortunately for her, she received a new heart and lungs. She happened to have bad lungs and they found for her a new heart and lung. I will be so grateful for that woman who said, I will give my heart out if you can get me a new heart and lung. What a decision to make. Thank God she made the right one. And her heart was made just for me.

And so we rejoiced together over this wonderful event in our lives and we praise God for it and people are willing to take a chance on an old guy with diabetes and an old guy who had a stroke and a few heart attacks and a few other things. And I spend my life now trying to find ways to help other people have a joy that I have in living with a brand new heart.

Thank you very much for your time.

[The prepared statement of Richard M. DeVos follows:]

PREPARED STATEMENT OF RICHARD M. DEVOS

I want to thank the Energy and Commerce Committee for giving me the opportunity to testify on the subject of "Assessing Initiatives to Increase Organ Donations." The subject of increasing organ donations is very close to my heart, and I feel very passionate about doing something to improve it. While years of deliberations have taken place, 16 patients die every day waiting for available organs that our present system fails to have donated. In their names, we should act now to correct this tragic failure of our system.

The key of our proposal is to shift the decision to the donor (Donor Authorization), as the previous speakers have proposed. Having been on the Board of the second largest donor hospital of deceased organs in the country and still missing a large number of possible donors, we became aware that when the patient's desires are known, almost always the organ donation follows. In the best American tradition, it is right that each individual make provisions to decide when they are able to participate in the decision of what is to be done with their organs in the event of brain death. This notion has finally taken hold in the transplant communities around the country and is now favored by many professional and family associations.

To be successful and access the 50% of the donor candidates that we are missing now, it will require the massive enrollment of millions of citizens. Educational campaigns, advertisements, enrollment drives, and all the methods tried up to now have yielded less than 40% of the population signing, where available, on the back of driver's licenses or donor cards, and proportionally even less people joining potential donor organizations.

For these reasons and based upon "Project Donor" of Gene Epstein and Al Boessmann, we propose to offer a $10,000 free term insurance-like benefit or a similar tax credit only to induce the individuals to sign the witnessed document when offered with the tax return form or driver's license application. These two activities reach almost 100% of the USA population at one time or another in their life. Why $10,000? Because it is an amount significant enough to make the individuals focus on the document offered and the designation of the after-death beneficiary of their generosity.

To address the right concerns of minorities that they would not be given adequate terminal care if an insurance or tax credit exists, this document can be accessed only when the patient has been declared brain dead and the family has been notified.

Each kidney transplanted alone saves between $200,000 and $400,000 to the insurers paying to keep these patients alive on the waiting list. Medicare pays 60% of these bills.

This proposal respects the autonomy of the individual, has been accepted by many diverse religious and ethical organizations, addresses the concern of minorities about their possible terminal care, empowers the poorer members of society to bequeath to their families the societal recognition of their generosity, and it makes economical sense, saving billions of dollars to the present payers.

Mr. GREENWOOD. That's what I would call straight talk.

Dr. Joseph Vacanti.

TESTIMONY OF JOSEPH P. VACANTI

Mr. VACANTI. Thank you, Mr. Chairman. I hope you analyze mine as well rather than gobbledygook. Thank you for the opportunity for me to testify today before this subcommittee.

I am a surgeon who practices pediatric surgery, as well as pediatric transplantation surgery. I have been in the practice of these two special areas of surgery in children since completing my training in 1983. My remarks today are in regard to the ever-increasing problem of vital organ shortages, and the work that I have done in trying to solve this problem.

As you are all aware, organ transplantation has been enormously successful and one of the major advances of 20th century medicine and surgery. However, it's this very success that has led to the ever-worsening problem of the organ donor shortage. We have all of the tools at our disposal of being successful in the transplantation of vital organs, but the fundamental thing we need is the vital organ itself. You have heard its numbers, over 80,000 Americans waiting, many die.

Now, this field that I represent, tissue engineering and regenerative medicine, has been developed to try and meet this need. Over the last 18 years, my laboratory, and many of my collaborators, have been developing technologies using biology, medicine and engineering to actually build these organs so that they're available on demand. This challenging and novel approach has advanced from fiction to reality. The work has now advanced into human therapy in several circumstances, but not yet for vital organs.

As an example, several commercially available skin products have been developed. In fact, the tragedy of September 11 produced many patients with horrible burn wounds. Tissue-engineered skin was donated to help these patients both survive and then have an improved quality of life. Besides skin, living cartilage, living bone, living blood vessels, and some early investigation into living human bladder are now available. The fundamental scientific and technologic basis of this approach has been developed over these past 18 years. There have been many new advances in the understanding of living cells and advances in material science to produce better and better living tissues. Given all this, the ultimate challenge is the creation of a life saving whole organ to solve the subject of this subcommittee.

Now, we continue to work on this most difficult problem at the Massachusetts General Hospital, Harvard, MIT and Draper Laboratories. Based on the work we have performed over the past 5 years, it is my feeling and my opinion that this problem is solvable and that the goal is achievable. It will require the firm commitment of intellectual resources for creative problem solving and financial resources to actually achieve the seemingly impossible. This year marks the 100th anniversary of the first human flight. All previous human civilizations had dreamed of human flight. However, it was American know-how and American determination that ultimately achieved this seemingly impossible goal 100 years ago. This new problem in biologic engineering can also be solved.

Thank you for the privilege of discussing this at this hearing.

[The prepared statement of Joseph P. Vacanti follows:]

PREPARED STATEMENT OF JOSEPH P. VACANTI, DIRECTOR, PEDIATRIC TRANSPLANTATION, MASSACHUSETTS GENERAL HOSPITAL, BOSTON

Thank you for the opportunity to testify today before the Subcommittee on Oversight and Investigations in the hearing "Assessing Initiatives to Increase Organ Donations".

I am a surgeon who practices pediatric surgery as well as pediatric transplantation surgery. I have been in the practice of these two special areas of surgery in children since completing my training in 1983. My remarks today are in regard to the ever increasing problem of vital organ shortages and the work that I have done in trying to solve this problem. As you all are aware, organ transplantation has been enormously successful and is one of the major advances of twentieth century medicine and surgery. However, its very success has led to the ever-worsening problem of organ donor shortage. We now have all of the tools at our disposal of being very successful in transplantation of vital organs. However, the fundamental thing we need is the vital organ for transplantation. Currently, there are over 80,000 Americans waiting for a vital organ to become available. The field of tissue engineering and regenerative medicine has been developed to try and meet this need. Over the last 18 years my laboratory with many of my collaborators have been developing technologies in biology, medicine, and engineering to actually make living tissues and organs for replacement therapy. This challenging and novel approach has advanced from fiction to reality. The work has now advanced into human therapy in several circumstances but not yet for vital organs. As an example, several commercially available skin products have been developed and commercialized. In fact, the tragic of September 11th produced many patients with horrible burn wounds. Tissue engineered skin was donated to help these patients both survive and then have an improved quality of life. Besides skin, products of living cartilage, living bone, living blood vessels, and some early investigation into living human bladder are now available.

The fundamental scientific and technologic basis of this approach has been developed over these past 18 years. There have been many new advances in the understanding of living cells and advances in material science to produce better and better living tissues.

Given all this, the ultimate challenge is the creation of a life-saving whole organ to solve the organ shortage. We continue to work on this most difficult problem at Harvard and the Massachusetts General Hospital, MIT, and the Draper Laboratories. Based on the work that we have performed over the past five years, it is my feeling that this problem is solvable and that the goal is achievable. It will require the firm commitment of intellectual resources for creative problem solving and financial resources to actually achieve the seemingly impossible. This year marks the 100th anniversary of the first powered human flight. All previous human civilizations had dreamed of human flight. However, it was American know-how and American determination that ultimately achieved this seemingly impossible goal 100 years ago. This new problem of biologic engineering can also be solved.

Thank you for the privilege of discussing this at this hearing.

Mr. GREENWOOD. Thank you. No gobbledygook at all. Rather straightforward.

Dr. Abraham Shaked.

TESTIMONY OF ABRAHAM SHAKED

Mr. SHAKED. Chairman Greenwood and distinguished members, thank you for the opportunity to submit this testimony on behalf of the American Society of Transplant Surgeons.

I am the Chief of Transplantation Surgery at the University of Pennsylvania and the Children's Hospital of Philadelphia. Myself, I have been an adult liver transplant surgeon. And if I may add a personal thing, it is going to be very exciting to come tonight and to tell my family and my children that I met you, Representative of our State. And one other thing about them, they all signed, by themselves, donor cards and God forbid something happens, our wishes will be respected.

This committee assesses the initiative to increase organ donation and would like to offer our comments on four different topics, two of them I would like to discuss in brief and two maybe a little bit more. In brief, we the American Society of Transplant Surgeons are a society of full transplant surgeons in this country including, by the way, Senator Frist, who is still a member and paying dues. We would like to offer our support for honoring donor wishes, what is referred in this country as donor rights. This is clearly something that should be supported, and we join other organizations in this initiative.

The second thing that we have to mention is the importance of research as mentioned by my friend Jay of research in this area. About a year ago or so, our society contributed about $2.1 million from a donation we had from members and the community to study, for example, what happened to donors and recipients after leaving donor liver transplantation. We did it with NIH. Our center is one of nine centers in the country studying this issue. And we truly believe that more research and what's going to come out from this NIH study is going to help citizens of our country, and we really thank you for support of the NIH in this initiative.

The two issues that I would like to expand a little bit more is the support for—the support for the use of organ coordinators in hospitals. And this—there is a lot of interest in this country on this issue. And a couple of years ago our society sponsored—we went to Spain for a couple of days, and we were able to spend some time with our great Spanish allies and we learned a lot from them and there is much to learn from that model. They were able to do something that should be done here. They were able to increase the number of donors per million, and they could show it to us clearly. And interestingly, there was an increase in all the donor population, and we used a lot of organs from these donors. And I think that is a nice thing to support. And we should provide some funds of some sort to initiate this model in this country. We think this is going to work, and we support legislation in this area.

Now, the other thing that we want to comment is this payment or incentive for donor organs and things like that. The ASTS is clearly opposed to payment for organs. And as a private citizen and as a representative of this organization, I have to say this was debated a lot, and we thought about it. This country has a lot of history—as a new immigrant to this country, I learned about the history here. This country has a lot of history in selling and buying human life. And there was a whole Civil War about it. And now we are talking about commercializing organs. This is not something that I think the culture in this country is ready for, and I hope will never be ready for.

However, there are all kinds of things that we should learn. And me as a scientist, I want to learn models, whether there is any opportunities to increase donations via project. One thing is for sure. We should never—not disincentivize the issue of donation. My family member was once a donor and it's terrible. You have to go there and spend time and to go back and forth. And there is more payment, believe it or not, for prepping the cadaver for viewing and all things coming out of pocket and the pocket is from the family and this should not be done. So we support projects to examine the issues. We may support projects to examine other issues that are acceptable and ethically acceptable and justified by our moral standards. And we want to do that in a scientific way, like what I do in my lab when I want to investigate, set up a model, see whether it's going this way or not and modify it so on and so forth. We think it should be studied in a careful way. Now, I understand there are a lot of restrictions within the law of how to do it and what to do. I am not a lawyer and I look at you, you are the leaders and you have to provide some kind of means or some kind of legal authority for us to study. At the same time you hold the money, and you should provide some kind of funds. We are there to conduct the study. We are there to provide you the results, and you should judge whether it's working or not.

Our society is engaged for quite awhile examining all models. We are willing to work with you at any time. Our problem is not to tell you how to change the law. That's what you're doing. That's your responsibility. Our responsibility is to provide you the results and to see whether it's working or not and we are there at any time.

And thanks very much.

[The prepared statement of Abraham Shaked follows:]

PREPARED STATEMENT OF ABRAHAM SHAKED, PRESIDENT, AMERICAN SOCIETY OF TRANSPLANT SURGEONS

Chairman Greenwood, Ranking Member Deutsch, and distinguished Members of the Subcommittee: On behalf of the American Society of Transplant Surgeons ("ASTS"), thank you for the opportunity to testify before this Subcommittee on the important issue of assessing initiatives to increase organ donation rates. My name is Abraham Shaked and I am Chief of Transplantation Surgery at the University of Pennsylvania, Department of Surgery.

Today marks my first day as President of ASTS, an organization comprised—of over 900 transplant surgeons dedicated to promoting and encouraging education and research with respect to organ and tissue transplantation so as to save lives and enhance the quality of life of patients with end stage organ failure. As this Subcommittee assesses initiatives to increase the rate of organ donation in this country, we would like to offer comments on four topics:

1. The use of organ coordinators in what is often referred to as the "Spanish model";
2. The ethical use of financial incentives to increase organ donation rates;
3. Honoring the donor's wishes, what is sometimes referred to a "donor rights"; and
4. The importance of living donor liver transplantation and related research.

BACKGROUND

Mr. Chairman, as you well know, one of the most pressing problems in the field of organ transplantation is the lack of available organ donors. This creates long waiting lists of potential candidates for organ transplants. Every individual who needs an organ transplant should be able to receive one in a timely manner but, as a nation, we are not even close to achieving this goal. The Bush Administration is providing strong leadership in this area, both in terms of funding of the programs under the Division of Transplantation within the Health Resources and Services Administration and with the assistance of his Advisory Committee on Transplantation

("ACOT"). Secretary Thompson, in particular, deserves great credit for his personal commitment to the organ donation issue. Along with a concerted effort in the transplant community and with the private sector, we are starting to turn the corner on this national problem, but there is much more progress to be made.

ASTS is very encouraged by the Bush administration's support for increased organ donation activities. In April 2001, Secretary of Health and Human Services Tommy Thompson first announced a five-point initiative to encourage organ, tissue, marrow, and blood donations. More recently, the Department of HHS has been working to implement the 18 recommendations of the ACOT. In past years, the third week in April was designated as "National Organ and Tissue Donor Awareness Week." This year, however, the Administration changed this to a month-long observance. Thousands of people have already recognized the importance of giving the "gift of life" to others. In 2002, 22,741 organ transplants and more than 46,000 corneal transplants were performed in the United States, and an average of 173 transplants were facilitated each month by the National Bone Marrow Donor Registry.

The need, however, is still enormous. Close to 81,000 individuals are on the waiting list for organ transplants, and thousands need tissue and corneal transplants each year. About 30,000 people per year are diagnosed with blood diseases that may be cured by a marrow/blood stem cell transplant. And each day, approximately 32,000 units of blood are needed, yet only about 5 percent of eligible blood donors give blood regularly.

Sadly, more than 6,000 people die unnecessarily each year because they did not receive the organ they needed. Currently, sixteen people die every day waiting for a donated organ—that is one death every 91 minutes. And the problem is getting worse, not better. Regrettably, in the past ten years, the number of registrations on the waiting list has quadrupled.

Mr. Chairman, there are many strategies to combat this problem, some more controversial than others. More often than not, simple awareness by patients and their families about the facts of organ donation can make the difference between life and death. Studies have shown that over 95% of families would consent to organ donation if they knew it was the wish of their loved one. As recent increases in organ donation rates demonstrate, education and awareness can be an effective tool in saving the lives of patients needing transplants. Consequently, the ASTS strongly favors initiatives that foster education and public awareness efforts. The commitment of federal resources to address the nationwide shortage of donated organs is essential to both increase the success rate in organ transplantation and increase the number of organ donors available.

While additional spending is critical on public awareness, grants for organ coordinators, grants for studies to eliminate disincentives to organ donation, and other programs, ASTS also supports changes in public policies to encourage donation. Several years ago, ASTS worked with a number of transplant-related organizations to craft a set of organ donation proposals for Secretary Thompson's consideration, and ultimately for the consideration of Congress. Now the bulk of these recommendations are represented in legislation introduced by Senate Majority Leader Bill Frist, who, as you know, is a transplant surgeon. This legislation, S.573, the "Organ Donation and Recovery Improvement Act," has widespread support and we hope to see it serve in the Senate as a vehicle to enact an organ donor bill into law this year.

THE USE OF ORGAN COORDINATORS

There has been significant U.S. interest in the potential promise that organ coordination programs, such as the program utilized in Spain, may offer. In fact, grants to fund organ coordination activities are proposed in Senator Frist's organ donation legislation, S. 573. In the House, Congressmen Wilson (R-SC) and Inslee (D-WA) have each sponsored similar legislation in the past. The so-called "Spanish Model" has been outlined as a structure of national, regional, and local or in-hospital efforts to increase organ donation. The management structure consists of a front-line in-hospital transplant coordinator who is fully involved and accountable for the donor recruitment effort. Furthermore, transplant donor coordination has been "professionalized" and most coordinators are qualified doctors, mainly intensive care specialists and nephrologists, who have dedicated time allocated to transplant coordination. Moreover, the Spanish system adheres to the principles of decentralization of the donor coordination effort through the use of regional coordinators and the establishment of organ procurement as the main priority for national, regional, and hospital coordinators.

In an attempt to assess and study whether organ coordination models could be effective for the U.S. in raising organ donation rates, the ASTS organized and funded a study group in the late 1990's to investigate methods of maximizing organ donor potential and improving the recovery of organs from these donors. The study group consisted of three transplant surgeons (John Roberts from the University of California San Francisco, Bruce Rosengard from the University of Pennsylvania, and myself as chair of the group) as well as four representatives from the Association of Organ Procurement Organizations (AOPO). The study group spent two days in Madrid, Spain at the Organizacion Nacional de Transplantes (ONT), that country's national transplant program.

Since the creation of the Organizacion Nacional de Trasplantes (ONT) in 1989, the organ donation rate in Spain has doubled. This effort has been so successful that it produced a 28% decrease in the size of the waiting list for kidney transplantation in Spain between 1991 and 1997. During this same time period, the US kidney waiting list nearly doubled in size. Although often attributed to improved donor recruitment efforts, the increase in donor rates in Spain may also represent higher utilization of marginal donors. Recently, a study examined age-related donor recruitment in Spain and the U.S. Chang, George J., MD, Mahanty, Harish D., MD, Ascher, Nancy L., MD PhD, Roberts, John P., MD, "Expanding the Donor Pool—Can the Spanish model work in the United States?" (Division of Transplantation, Department of Surgery, University of California, San Francisco).

Data from the ONT, the US Scientific Registry of Transplant Recipients (SRTR), the US Census Bureau, and the Tempus databank of Spain's Instituto Nacional de Estadistica (INE) were analyzed. Between 1989-1999, the number of donors in Spain increased from 14.3 to 33.7 per million population (pmp), (136% increase) compared to an increase in the US from 16.2 to 21.5 donors pmp (33%). The largest difference between Spain and the US in the increased number of donors was in the 45 year old group representing 30.3% of donors in Spain in 1999 (44 donors pmp). If the U.S. increased its older donor rates to match Spain's, an incremental 1235 donors per year would be realized. The high Spanish organ donation rates are largely attributable to increased use of older donors. Utilizing similar proportions of older donors in the US would increase the donor pool by almost 40%.

As already stated, there has been significant interest in implementing a "Spanish Model" for organ donation in the US and other countries. Calls for funding similar types of organizational structures have been made on the grounds that this change will result in an increase in organ availability. ASTS supports legislation that would create such organ coordination programs in the U.S. and believes that such a model can be effective, along with the practice of expanding the donor pool by utilizing older donors.

THE ETHICAL USE OF FINANCIAL INCENTIVES TO INCREASE ORGAN DONATION

The use of financial incentives to increase organ donation rates can be quite controversial and, of course, payment for organs is prohibited by current law under the National Organ Transplant Act (NOTA). NOTA prohibits the exchange of "valuable consideration" for the use of a person's organs. 42 U.S.C. 274e. To do so would run the risk of turning what is now often referred to as the "gift of life" into a commodity to be bought and sold. This potentially cheapens the sanctity of human life and raises profound moral, ethical and religious questions. These questions, however, must be weighed against the morality of tolerating huge organ donor waiting lists with thousands of people dieing each year unnecessarily.

The ASTS clearly opposes payment for organs. The United States must not send a signal to the international "black market" that the United States tolerates the commoditization of human organs. However, ASTS does not oppose efforts to study various methods and programs to increase donation rates that may have a financial component. For instance, ASTS would support a demonstration project that assessed the effectiveness of providing a modest funeral expense benefit to the family of a decedent donor, not as a payment for a donated organ, but as a token of thanks. ASTS also supports initiatives to eliminate financial disincentives to donation such as the provision of travel and subsistence expenses for living donors and similar initiatives.

Mr. Chairman, ASTS is well aware of your bill introduced in the 107th Congress, H.R. 5224, that addressed the issue of financial incentives without permitting such incentives to override the provisions of NOTA. Senator Frist's bill in this Congress, S. 573, takes a slightly different approach by stating that demonstration projects on financial incentives may be conducted "Notwithstanding [the provisions] of NOTA..." This language appears to open the door to financial incentive demonstration projects that may not be considered permissible under current law. However, Senator Frist's bill contains two important provisions that help ensure that such demonstrations will be ethically sound before being funded by the Department of

Health and Human Services. First, the Secretary is required to submit a report to Congress before funding any initiatives that evaluates "the ethical implications of proposals for demonstration projects to increase cadaveric donation."

Second, the bill requires the Secretary to provide "ongoing ethical review and evaluation." While ASTS would prefer that this review be provided by an entity that is independent from HHS, such as the President's Council on Bioethics, and will continue to work in the Senate to accomplish this goal, ASTS supports S. 573 and looks forward to the day that an organ donation bill will be signed into law.

ASTS SUPPORTS DONOR RIGHTS

ASTS recently formally endorsed a policy of honoring donor wishes in the donation decision, notwithstanding familial objections. This policy is consistent with current federal law but many states are currently considering "donor rights" laws of their own. Formal endorsements of donor rights by AOPO and the Advisory Committee on Transplantation preceded ASTS's decision, all of which have occurred in the last several weeks. It is ASTS' hope that raising the awareness level of donor rights will have an impact on the number of people who take affirmative steps to witness their intent to donate their organs upon death.

ASTS AND NIH PARTNERSHIP

ASTS and the NIH have a solid history of partnering on projects that will increase the rates of organ donation, improve existing transplant protocols, and provide basic research into transplantation. This year, the NIH announced, in coordination with ASTS, the *Adult to Adult Living Donor Liver Transplant Cohort Study* (A2ALL), to take place at 10 U.S. transplant centers over the next seven years. ASTS has committed over $2.1 million over a seven year period for this joint project. The national project will investigate the experience of a group of patients eligible for living donor liver transplantation, focusing on the factors influencing outcomes of living donor liver transplants for both donors and recipients. Researchers will compare outcomes of this new procedure with the outcomes for patients who receive donor livers from cadavers.

The goal of the study is to gather accurate data in a disciplined, careful way so that liver transplant patients and potential donors have reliable information about the risks and benefits of living organ donation. In addition to vital clinical issues, the A2ALL will investigate important research issues such as liver regeneration, liver cancer, and infectious hepatitis.

Liver transplantation is the only cure and a life-saving measure for people with end-stage liver disease. Although liver transplants have become relatively common in the U.S. in recent decades, in 2001 some 17,000 patients waited for livers to be donated, while fewer than 5,000 cadaveric livers were actually transplanted that year. The shortage of cadaveric organs has led physicians and researchers to look to live donors to close that gap. The liver is a large segmented organ that can potentially be split without harm to the donor and with benefit to the recipient. Because the liver, unlike most organs, has a remarkable ability to regenerate, the donor's remaining liver grows to its original size within weeks. Likewise, the donated lobe will also grow in the recipient's body.

For children in need of liver transplantation, living donor transplantation from an adult has been very successful and has become an accepted medical option. Adults in need of liver transplantation require a larger segment, as much as half or more of the donor's liver. This requires a more extensive and complex surgery, with potentially greater risks for the donor and the recipient. The procedure has evolved so rapidly that over half of the living donor transplants performed to date have occurred since 2000. Evaluation of donors as well as surgical procedures vary from one transplant center to another. Although the large majority of living donor liver transplants have been successful, there are few data to inform potential donors about risks. Post-surgical problems for donors can include infection, pneumonia, and leaking bile, which can require further surgery.

Because the procedure is expanding across the country, a group of concerned physicians recently called for more research on the risks and benefits of this procedure as well as an outside regulator to certify hospitals that would perform the procedure in the New England Journal of Medicine (April 4, 2002). They also asked for uniform medical criteria in selecting donors and recipients.

Mr. Chairman, transplant surgeons place a great deal of importance on the well-being of both donors and recipients. ASTS's partnership with NIDDK should give us credible data for the high quality patient care we all want to provide.

CONCLUSION

Thank your, Mr. Chairman, for the opportunity to present the views of the ASTS before this Subcommittee. Please do not hesitate to contact me in the future if I can be of any further assistance. Thank you.

Mr. GREENWOOD. Thank you.

Dr. Delmonico.

TESTIMONY OF FRANCIS L. DELMONICO

Mr. DELMONICO. Thank you.

I am Francis Delmonico. I am a transplant surgeon of 25 years, Medical Director of the New England Organ Bank. I am a member of the Secretary's Advisory Committee on Transplantation. And I am honored to represent the National Kidney Foundation, and thank you for having this opportunity to appear before you.

The NKF acknowledges the support of Congress previously about disincentives for live donors to be donors and that ought not to be. So I wish to acknowledge, on behalf of the NKF, the passage of the Organ Donation Improvement Act of 2003. This kind of mind-set, to say to people we shouldn't have them bear the expenses of being a live donor, is very important, but that is clearly different than saying someone's going to step forward to be a donor by the motivation of being monetarily enriched. So that is an ethical distinction I would hope that you would really take into consideration. The NOTA of 1984 prohibits anyone from acquiring and transferring, as has been stated this morning, a human organ for valuable consideration.

The NKF supports this legislation. In fact, so do all the folks who have been here this morning. We know them personally, and they have called the caution of overruling that in the following sense, that now the reason someone comes forward is a valuable consideration by money or property. That is a very important ethical distinction, and it goes to the payments of organs. That would be the headline as it would come if there were these financial incentives applied. Payments do the following; they exploit vulnerable members of society. And that degree of exploitation, I would say to you, as we now know from the black market around the world of organ sales, is influenced by where they live, by their gender, by their ethnicity, by their social status. That is a reality that is well-described.

So to suggest that the Congress now is going to endorse financial incentives, please, if I may respectfully say, think through what the impact of that headline will be, payments for organs. That then, in a State such as Michigan or some locale where is there a demonstration project that you wish to have that financial incentive applied, please don't have it perceived that the Federal or State government is the proprietor of an organ sale which could be misconstrued, which are the headlines that are taking place now, when these kinds of financial incentives are being proposed, because that will have an impact around the world as if to say, there's a sanction now for a market for organs and it's impossible.

Once you get into that market to say, well, we will have it government regulated around the world, I don't think so. Another piece of this, if I might say this personally, I had an opportunity to debate a columnist at the University of Chicago a week ago, a

Nobel lawyer, a bit over my head academically, but his posture was that in a global economy, we might be able to import individuals to sell their kidney. And then the question was, and then the NKF would have this question as well, when we are done selling a kidney, can she sell a part of her liver, or then can there be the sale of the lung. So where do the sales stop? Where does the element of coercion and exploitation not be the overriding concern.

There is another aspect of this that I would like to bring to the committee's attention as a transplant surgeon. Advocacy for organ vendors presents an inherent conflict in the physician's relationship with the patient. I have a donor before me now. I have had this for 25 years. Now, put money in the mix of that equation. How are they going to trust my medical decisionmaking, that this person should be a donor or not if there are medical reasons why that are not medically suitable? Think of the patient coming before me saying, "I need the $40,000. You have got to enable me to be a donor, no matter what the medical problem might be." Let's say there is a medical history of cancer or some medical contraindication, will that surface in the mix of that patient-physician relationship? I would only bring to you a very ernest concern about that trust and relationship.

Organ sellers around the world know the difference of this, and there have been reports in the literature regarding the consequences of being a black marketed organ seller and the difficulties that these individuals have had. So now you get into financial incentives and you are applying, arbitrarily, a monetary assignment for this. Well, the difficulty of this becomes will we throw $10,000 at it, and does that not become a way of evaluating the very human life that all of us at this table have had for all of our years.

The proponents of financial incentives for nonliving organ donation assert that demonstration projects should be conducted to determine whether it will increase the organ supply. The concern the NKF has is that the headline will be payment for organs and that it's impossible to distinguish that financial incentive for nonliving donation from this practice that we just elaborated about selling human organs. The experience of this goes to the integrity of the organ donor pool, as well as paid blood donations.

I would say to you, another factor of this, that the NKF has been confronted with is that it will undermine the good, the altruism that has been by half of the donors who have come forward and not been compensated. So in the interest of time, let me say the NKF— that the medical community commends what we have heard this morning from Dr. Metzger and Joe Roth and this opportunity to honor the potential organ donors' wishes. The notion of the decedent's self-determination not being overruled and yet at the same time, I know the NKF wishes to underscore that while fulfilling donors' wishes, the OPO staff and hospital staff must be sensitive to the needs of the families at that time of crisis.

So on the one hand, we are propelling donor authorization and donor rights, but at the same time let us not overlook the families that are there in their time of crisis. So this approach of honoring donor wishes which is the thrust behind the Uniform Anatomical Gift Act—and by the way, as a member of the ACOT we wrote—

we endorsed this at the ACOT—a wonderful development. We would hope that you would consider that very seriously and work with ways to see that becomes endorsed and implemented joining the entire transplant community to embrace a social responsibility about organ donation, rather than say we'll throw money to it. This is an alternative approach. And I would say to you, rather than the perception of a financial incentive to be buying and selling of organs, that would derive an ethical consensus that I think we could all devote ourselves to.

[The prepared statement of Francis L. Delmonico follows:]

PREPARED STATEMENT OF FRANCIS DELMONICO, NATIONAL KIDNEY FOUNDATION

Good Morning. I am Francis Delmonico, a transplant surgeon at Massachusetts General Hospital, Professor of Surgery at Harvard Medical School, and a volunteer for the National Kidney Foundation (NKF), as a member of the NKF's Medical and Scientific Advisory Board. On behalf of the 30,000 members of the NKF, including several thousand solid organ transplant recipients, we appreciate the opportunity to present testimony today.

The NKF acknowledges the support that Congress has provided for organ donation in legislation to assist living organ donors with non-medical expenses such as travel and subsistence, which is included in the recent House passage of H.R. 399, the "Organ Donation Improvement Act of 2003." Surveys of living kidney donors conducted by the NKF have revealed that 1 in 4 respondents experienced a burden with non-reimbursed expenses. We are encouraged that H.R. 399 will enhance the opportunity for live organ donation.

Remuneration of expenses related to donation, whether living or non-living, is ethically different than a monetary payment that enriches a person as the motivation to be an organ donor. The National Organ Transplant Act (NOTA) of 1984 prohibits anyone from acquiring, receiving, or transferring a human organ for valuable consideration for use in human transplantation. The NKF supports this legislation because the sale of bodies or body parts would undermine the fundamental values of our society. Payments would exploit the most vulnerable members of our society, with the degree of exploitation influenced by gender, ethnicity, and the social status of the vendor. This exploitation has been the experience of a black market for organs throughout the world. To suggest that the Federal Government or individual States be the proprietor of a market for organs is contrary to the proper role of government. For those global economists who would import a poor person into this country even for the noble reason to feed her family by selling her kidney, the NKF would ask: will these market forces next suggest that our government sanction her selling a part of her liver, then a lobe of her lung?

Advocacy for organ vendors (versus donors) also presents an inherent conflict for the physician's professional relationship with a patient. In that relationship, patients are not clients, nor commodities. It should be evident that money as a motivation for "donation" distorts the basis of the physician patient relationship: the trust of each other. The medical decision and procedure that may be forced upon the organ seller and the physician are not by the priority of best care, but rather by the dictate of the sale.

Organ sellers are now reported to know the difference between a proper patient-physician relationship and the complicated interaction they have experienced, much to their regret. These unfortunate individuals are not considered as patients but objects of an arbitrary monetary calculation, driven by the going rate in the market place (government regulated or not). Any attempt to assign a monetary value to the human body or its body parts, even in the hope of increasing organ supply, diminishes human dignity and devaluates the very human life we seek to save.

Proponents of financial incentives for non-living organ donation assert that demonstration projects should be conducted to determine whether it will increase the organ supply. However, the NKF believes that it is impossible to separate the ethical debate of financial incentives for non-living donation from the unethical practice of selling human organs. Payments for organs could undermine the integrity of the organ donor pool as was the experience of paid blood donations. Furthermore, the advocates of such demonstration projects have given no formula as to how they will make a distinction of endorsing live donor sales, nor have they assured appropriate ethical oversight to prevent potential donor families from perceiving this project as merely a payment for organs.

For demonstration projects of financial incentives to be initiated in the United States, it will require a revision of the federal law by Congress. The consequence of a congressional endorsement of a payment for organs would be profound. It could propel other countries to sanction an unethical and unjust standard of immense proportions, one in which the wealthy readily obtain organs from the poor, justified by the citation of congressional sanction. In that reality, the poor person will remain poor but lose health and maybe more than one organ in the process of a government authorized abuse of the poor for the rich.

Opposition to payment for organs is not limited to the NKF. The American College of Surgeons has said that compensation of any kind for organs is wrong. The President of The American Society of Transplant Surgeons (ASTS) has testified this morning that the ASTS opposes payments for living or deceased organs.

What can we all do now to increase deceased organ donation beyond recent efforts? The NKF commends the approach brought to the Committee's attention today by Robert Metzger of the United Network for Organ Sharing (UNOS) in concert with Joe Roth representing the Association of Organ Procurement Organizations (AOPO): to honor the potential organ donor's wishes. What better way could a mournful family reconcile some of its grief, than to honor their loved one's desire to provide an altruistic gift to individuals in need? The decedent's self determination to donate should not be overruled. However, the NKF also wishes to underscore that while fulfilling donor wishes, the OPO and hospital staff must be sensitive to the needs of families at the time of crisis. The NKF supports the needs and expectations of donor families through its National Donor Family Council (NDFC), which we founded in 1992. With more than 10,000 donor family and professional members, the NDFC represents donors of all organs and tissues.

This approach of honoring the donor's wishes was the thrust behind the Uniform Anatomical Gift Act (UAGA) promulgated in every state many years ago and recently endorsed by the Secretary of Health's Advisory Committee on Transplantation. Thus, the NKF joins today with the all of the transplant community to create a timely national momentum to embrace a social responsibility conveyed by the donor authorization initiative. The NKF affirms the right of individuals to authorize the donation of their organs and tissues at death. This alternative approach to buying and selling organs brings an ethical consensus to which we all can devote ourselves.

Thank you. I would be pleased to respond to any questions.

Mr. GREENWOOD. The Chair recognizes himself for 10 minutes, and we have heard the spectrum of views on this issue.

Let me direct a question right back to you, Dr. Delmonico, if I may, because you had indicated that something to the effect that it would be impossible to distinguish between financial incentives that went to a decedent's estate versus buying an organ from a living person and creating that incentive. And I want to challenge that assertion, because I think people don't have a lot of difficulty making discrimination between someone who is alive and someone who is dead. And, obviously, since no one that I am aware of is advocating a policy that would actually pay someone to donate a kidney while they are alive, I think that is ethically abhorrent to all of us. You are putting that person's life at risk. And what I understand, it is more dangerous to live with one kidney than with two. So that would be financial incentive that would put someone at significant risk. But when someone is making a decision whether or not to sign up to be a donor, this is not something that is occurring at the moment—this is not when they're on their death bed or not at a moment when they're anticipating this would actually happen to them. Most people know when they sign up to be an organ donor, it is very unlikely that they will be one. Takes very special circumstances to be an appropriate donor. So I don't see—your testimony talks a lot about the blurring of this distinction, that somehow that even if we had a study program in which there would be some kind of financial remuneration to an individual's estate or to a charity of an individual's choice upon their death, that that would incentivize black market organ donation in China. And I don't see the slope as being slippery in that regard. And when I take into consideration the ethics of allowing 6,000 people to die every year, it's a pretty extraordinary value to put on one side of the scale, 6,000 lives when we're talking about some kind of mild incentive. We heard talk about $5 off on your driver's license. That is a financial incentive. I don't see anyone screaming about that and arguing that people are selling their organs or headlines are blurring the distinction.

Mr. DELMONICO. Could I respond to that, please?

We agree we have got to get people to sign up. You have expressed this morning your desire to do this in such a way that it applies to a financial incentive. The issue is—now, I am saying this respectfully—how do you go about it.

Mr. GREENWOOD. Of course.

Mr. DELMONICO. I had the experience—I am a member of the American Society of Transplant Surgeons. They asked that the Ethics Committee address this issue. We did. And the conclusion was that there should be a study, and perhaps with the use of a funeral reimbursement, the headline read, Surgeons Endorse Payments for Organs in the Washington Post. The Society was understandably quite concerned that there was the wrong perception. It is by that experience that I wish for you—only that I respectfully say, one has to be careful about how this is perceived because once it goes to the Federal Government and endorses payments for organs by such a financial incentive or a particular State does, then I don't see how you rein that in throughout the world.

So it's by that experience that I express that concern, but we both agree, let's get folks to sign up.

Mr. GREENWOOD. But if I may, it seems to me that for the years that I have been interested in this subject, everything—I have heard that a thousand times, let's get more people to sign up and yet we have a flat line. Nothing has made a significant dent in the number of donors.

Mr. DELMONICO. Yes, sir. But Dr. Metzger's approach has not been tried, and that's the best way I can respond. We are both wanting the same objective to have people sign up. It's just a matter of how we go about getting them to do it.

Mr. GREENWOOD. We need to be extraordinarily careful, and I think Dr. Sade as he went through the precautions that need to be taken, was very clear about how this needs to be done.

And if you would respond to Dr. Delmonico on the question of whether or not this can be done in an ethically appropriate way and in a way that doesn't produce the unintended consequences that he fears.

Mr. SADE. Well, the short answer is, yes, indeed, it can be done in an ethically appropriate way. That is financial incentives can be used in ethically appropriate ways. I would like to make a couple of comments about several of the speakers so far. We heard them talk about putting money into the equation as far as donations are concerned, places a value on human life and somehow this doesn't feel right and this is repugnant in some way. Well, the other side of that is, they are also putting a value on human life of the potential recipients who will never get those organs and the value in that case is very low. It's not very valuable at all. Well, I beg to differ with that. I think that the lost lives are very important.

Also, I personally don't worry very much about headlines. I worry more about 6,000 people dying every year. There were lots of big headlines about all kinds of issues in the past. For example, in vitro fertilization was terribly controversial and people yelled and screamed about how unethical it is and how terrible it is. That made headlines. Today there are thousands of woman every year who benefit from in vitro fertilization and have children that they never could have had otherwise.

So I am not concerned about headlines. We can get past those. I think that the first business of physicians and Federal legislation in supporting the health care system is to make sure that as many patients live as possible within the boundaries of ethical behavior and ethical means. And there's no reason why we can't design studies that meet ethical standards that do involve financial incentives.

Mr. GREENWOOD. I would like ask Mr. DeVos to respond to Dr. Shaked or Dr. Delmonico who obviously have a different point than you do with regard to financial incentives.

Mr. DEVOS. Dr. Delmonico and I have visited and I respect him greatly. I am hardly in a league to even talk because of his position and his experience. I am just a guy on the other end of the list, and so I look at it from if I wanted a new knee, they would pay for a new knee. I mean I would pay for that. I mean the idea that we came up with and your guys in Philadelphia—your guys in Pennsylvania came up with, find a way around rewarding and buying and selling organs, which was let's just put some money in, the idea of getting somebody to sign. It's a reward for signing a card. It has nothing to do with use of the organs ultimately. It does because it ends up that way, but of the millions that we need, only a few thousand will end up there, and most of them will die.

Mr. DEVOS. But nevertheless we have got to get those millions to sign. And if a stiff—and if 10 bucks will do it, fine. But if I'm talking to a bunch of college kids, and I say, "Hey, we will put 10,000 into your estate if you do this," they might say, "Yeah, that's okay. I'll go do that." Well, that's all we're looking for. This is an encouragement, like an automobile discount. I know that's pretty crude for these people, but, you know from a business guy's standpoint, those are incentives people offer to get people to do things.

And so all this is, is incentive to get people to do things. I respect their fears. Those are all great fears. And so we've got to find a way to do this to where we package it correctly and present it correctly. It is a payment for the act of signing a card. That's all it is. It's nothing more than that. And if we can keep that there, maybe we can get this done. All I want to do is get more organs, and I want to do it ethically and all. But if I'm a guy waiting on the list, I'm not quite as concerned about all the other things that might happen somewhere else in the world as I am about, how about a heart for me, guy?

Mr. GREENWOOD. Thank you. It seems to me there's a three-step process here. You'd have to design some kind of a system, and then you'd have to pilot program it, and then you'd have to see whether it's worth expanding or not.

My time has expired. I'm just going to ask Dr. Sade, very briefly, has anyone—you talked about the need to set this up in a way that would be ethical and have an IRB? Is there a design on paper that meets those tests yet, whether we change the law or not?

Mr. SADE. Not as far as I know. Not the specific tests that we have suggested. There have been suggestions for various kinds of financial incentives that make a lot of sense.

Pennsylvania offered to pay for funeral expenses. The delegation from Utah presented a bill a couple of years ago, 3 years ago to allow a $10,000 tax benefit in inheritance taxes. And talking about poor people being—the focus of organ donation. That would actually focus at the higher end of the economic spectrum. Studies could be designed in a number of ways that could spread the donation of organs over the—over a wide range of the population.

Mr. GREENWOOD. My time has expired. The gentlelady from Colorado.

Ms. DEGETTE. Thank you, Mr. Chairman.

Mr. DeVos I do appreciate your can-do attitude. However, I don't think that there is one single person who's testified today who would equate organ donation to an automobile discount, and I think we all need to understand that.

I do have a question for you though, and here's my question. In your testimony, you state, and I'm quoting verbatim, to address the right concerns of minorities, that they would not be given adequate terminal care if an insurance or tax credit exists. This document can be accessed only when the patient has been declared brain dead and the family has been notified. That's your written testimony, right? Here's my question. Why is it you single out minorities for this concern? And wouldn't white people and everybody have that same concern?

Mr. DEVOS. Yes, I think so.

Ms. DEGETTE. So why did you just say minorities in your testimony?

Mr. DEVOS. I don't know. They stuck it in here, and I——

Ms. DEGETTE. Who's they?

Mr. DEVOS. They thought, well, because of the people who object always that it's a class issue, and so my doctor, who I work with, you know——

Ms. DEGETTE. Who put the word minority in there?

Mr. DEVOS. All the objections we get is on class distinctions about who would be——

Ms. DEGETTE. Now, some minorities are rich, right. I mean not all minorities are poor. It's a class issue, not a race issue, right?

Mr. DEVOS. To me, this is, you know——

Ms. DEGETTE. It's not a racial issue really. It's a class issue that you're trying to do, right?

Mr. DEVOS. Well, I don't know. It's only an issue of people who are concerned about this.

Ms. DEGETTE. And you think that's minorities?

Mr. DEVOS. That will give somebody an incentive to take my life to get an organ because then I would be incentivized by that.

Ms. DEGETTE. Okay. Dr. Sade, I'm wondering if you have any idea how many people in this country have volunteered to donate their organs either through drivers' license programs or other kinds of organ donations programs.

Mr. SADE. Yeah, it's very difficult to get a precise count of that, but the best estimates that I've seen are under 20 percent probably.

Ms. DEGETTE. In numbers of Americans, how many numbers of Americans? Would it be in the——

Mr. SADE. Fifteen percent of the adult population.

Ms. DEGETTE. So in the millions of people?

Mr. SADE. It's in the millions of people.

Ms. DEGETTE. And the organ shortfall in this country, as everybody's been saying, is around 6,000 people? Around 6,000 people die per year because they don't get a donated organ, right?

Mr. SADE. That's correct.

Ms. DEGETTE. And so what we're talking about is increasing it from the millions of Americans who've already agreed to donate organs to some more millions of Americans in the hopes, essentially, that we can find those 6,000 organs plus more, right?

Mr. SADE. Yes.

Ms. DEGETTE. Okay. Now, under what the AMA has been thinking about, who would the financial incentives go to, the donor or the donor's family?

Mr. SADE. That would depend on how the study is designed. The AMA has not recommended any particular form of financial incentive. What we're recommending is that financial incentives be designed according, in accord with the ethos, the mores of, the opinions of the population in which the study is going to be carried out.

Ms. DEGETTE. The reason I'm asking this question is because I asked the previous panel, and I think Mr. Greenwood's idea is that the financial incentives would go to the donor. But you don't have any particular opinion. So under what the AMA is thinking, there could be a study designed where someone is lying there in the hospital, and the doctor would come to their family and say, "Okay, we'll give you a $10,000 death benefit if you donate the organs." Could that be a possibility of a study?

Mr. SADE. I doubt that that would be—that such a study would be designed.

Ms. DEGETTE. And why?

Mr. SADE. Because there would be a great deal of feeling, as you're expressing very clearly, against it.

Ms. DEGETTE. Right. I agree. And I think appropriately so, don't you?

Mr. SADE. Perhaps. I'm willing to listen to any possibility that a group of investigators, in accord with the population that they wish to study, have agreed upon.

Ms. DEGETTE. Okay.

Mr. SADE. I'm not going to impose my values on a different section of the country.

Ms. DEGETTE. Okay. It sounds to me like the AMA hasn't settled on one type of study here. They just think it'd be a good idea to study, right?

Mr. SADE. To study a variety of different kinds of incentives; that's correct.

Ms. DeGette. Okay. Because how would this study be designed? Would there be a limited, well-defined experiment with a tight protocol? Or would there be a general repeal of the ban to allow all of these different things to happen?

Mr. Sade. Oh, no. What we would envision, and I don't know that this is the way it would happen, is that there would be waivers for a specific demonstration project for example.

Ms. DeGette. And who would give those waivers the HHS?

Mr. Sade. Well, the waivers would have to come through Congress because it's a national law.

Ms. DeGette. So Congress—so suddenly, Mr. Greenwood and I would be deciding?

Mr. Greenwood. Will the lady yield?

Ms. DeGette. I'd be happy to yield. Maybe you can clear it up.

Mr. Greenwood. I think the theory is that we would amend the law so that it would still remain illegal, in general, to provide incentives, but it would give the Secretary of Health and Human Services the opportunity to approve very limited pilot projects pursuant to the language that we would use in the legislation.

Ms. DeGette. Okay. So maybe I can ask the chairman then, would one of the studies that might be allowed be financial incentives to the families of the potential donors? Because the AMA seems to think we should explore everything.

Mr. Greenwood. If the gentlelady would yield again.

Ms. DeGette. Be happy to.

Mr. Greenwood. I think it seems obvious to me that we would— that no one would ever want to do anything that would create that kind of an adverse situation. Nobody wants to see, certainly not this Member of Congress, and I don't think any of our witnesses would think it would be appropriate to provide a financial incentive for a family to make a decision about a member of that family based on their financial consideration. That would be ethically abhorrent and neither the Congress nor the Secretary of Health and Human Services should approve such a thing.

Ms. DeGette. Reclaiming my time, Dr. Sade, do you have any idea how the study would be limited? Would it be limited by type of organ? Initially?

Mr. Sade. That depends on the people who design the study.

Ms. DeGette. Okay. So you don't have any—the AMA has no view on that.

Mr. Sade. No specific view; that's correct.

Ms. DeGette. Would it be limited by area of the country?

Mr. Sade. As far as the AMA is concerned, any area of the country that desires to carry out such a study would be welcome to do so. The more data we have, the more we know, and the more intelligent decisions we can make.

Ms. DeGette. So you could have a variety of studies, maybe a whole State would do one thing and one study maybe one of the transplantation centers would do it by organ. The AMA hasn't settled on one type of study?

Mr. Sade. Absolutely. I think that the kind of diversity of investigation that you're talking about is exactly what we would be after. We need information. We need data because we can't make intelligent well-informed decisions about what is ethical, what works, what doesn't work without information that tells us what the harms are and what the benefits are.

Ms. DeGette. Okay. But, see, here's the thing. In your testimony, you said that the AMA proposes that IRBs would oversee the types of studies, right?

Mr. Sade. The function of the IRB is to assure that certain processes are followed in protecting the human subjects and that sort of thing.

Ms. DeGette. But how do you that, when you haven't narrowed down what type of study you're going to do? Let me give you an example. The reason I asked you how many have signed organ donor forms, I've done some work with IRBs and usually what happens is an IRB approves a study that's going to be targeted at one type of patient. So for example, in the diabetes context, let's say you're doing an islet cell transplantation. You have defined subjects. You have defined human subjects, and the study protocol says we're going to use these types of patients and here's what we're going to do. What you have here is, you have incentives that you're trying to get people who you don't know to be organ donors, to agree to be organ donors. How's that going to work? How are you going to have an IRB approving that kind of study? I don't think there's any precedent for that.

Mr. Sade. I think what you are describing is the role of an IRB in the evaluation and approval or disapproval of a randomized clinical trial. That's not what we're dealing with here. We're dealing with a much—with a different kind of research project and IRBs deal with those. They just make sure that all of the rules that are part of the common—that come from the common rule, as well as their own local rules regarding how human subjects are handled in research, are followed. And they put a stamp of approval or not, depending on the design of the study and whether certain guidelines have been followed. They can do more than look at randomized clinical trials.

Ms. DeGette. With all due respect, sir, I think that some of the kinds of studies you're talking about would be perfectly appropriate for IRB approval. Other kinds I think would be far too generalized to even begin to come up with a protocol. And the thing I'm worried about, and, you know, Mr. Greenwood and I fight a lot of battles together, and we hardly fight any battles against each other, but sometimes we do. What I'm concerned about is that in essence, to do these kinds of studies—the AMA's thinking is so broad here that we would, in essence, have to repeal the ban in order to make this happen. And I'm very concerned about this for many of the reasons some of the witnesses talked about.

And if I may, Mr. Chairman, let me just ask unanimous consent for an additional 30 seconds.

Mr. Greenwood. Barely because we're going to have a vote any minute, and I want the gentleman from Oregon to have his opportunity.

Ms. DeGette. We've had lots of experts testify today. We've only had three people testify who have had direct involvement with the United States transplantation system. Mr. DeVos had his transplant abroad because he was ineligible here. All of those people said these kinds of decisions are very personal decisions, and they don't think financial incentives work. I'm all for working with you and everybody here on increasing the number of donors and increasing the number of organ transplant donors, but I don't think financial incentives is the way to go, and I think this is so broadly construed that it would have PR problems, but more importantly, it would have great ethical concerns.

So I look forward to working with you, and I thank you for your comity and the extra time.

Mr. GREENWOOD. The Chair thanks the gentlelady, and looks forward to working getting on the same page with you. And I have no doubts that we will.

The gentleman from Oregon.

Mr. WALDEN. I appreciate the confidence my chairman just expressed about getting on the same page with my colleague and friend from Colorado. Hope blossoms eternal.

Mr. DeVos, if my recollection serves me right, you've had some level of experience in creating organizations that motivate people to do things, is that not——

Mr. DEVOS. Well, I hope so.

Mr. WALDEN. A little organization called Amway?

Mr. DEVOS. I built a little company that motivates people all over the world. I keep trying to find ways. I do it with recognition, rewards and money. And they all work for different people.

Mr. WALDEN. Recognition, rewards and money. And do you—do you share the ethical concerns that have been raised? If you could develop a system that would work, would you apply it to live donors as well as to dead donors or dying donors?

Mr. DEVOS. I wasn't ever thinking of live donors because that's kind of a new thing, I think. And I think it requires a whole different set of thought and conditioning. You know, my experiences where I come from as a guy waiting and given new life, and I just said what can I do to help more people do that. So I'm kind of a simplistic soul in this deal. I like money and most people like money. And I look at it simply. She's got it all complicated, and I guess if you start from—you're opposed to the principle of it, then you look at all those things, and those are all legitimate things you have to look at. I was just saying, hey if I got a bunch of people and I want to motivate them—I love reward. I love the altruistic idea of giving it. I wish everybody in America would work for the love of work. But they seem to get moved by getting a little incentive. And our incentive has got nothing to do with the family. We've removed it totally from the family. It's all over on the signing of the card, so that when they get to the hospital, it's an automatic deal. Nobody has to be traumatic about it. Oh, I hate to do this. And I have listened to those people who wish they had when they didn't. And I've been hanging around this crowd for 6 years now. So it's kind of new for me, not technically, but all I know is my frustration has stopped. So all I want to say is, hey, I think there's—find us some way to get some young people to do it altruistically for some. We've got a lot of people signing, but that flat line bothered me, and I just said, well, let's try money. We tried reward, recognition. Let's try a little money and see what happens.

Mr. WALDEN. Is that the flat line on donations or the potential flat line on an EKG that bothered you the most?

Mr. DEVOS. Both ways. It's the flat line. We haven't been able to increase donations in 5 years. I hang around with the people at Mayo and all these places, and they all are complaining and closing because they don't get enough organs. So those—I said, well, let's try something new.

Mr. WALDEN. I appreciate that. And I obviously share the concern that you had about trying to get people to donate. And I certainly, from obviously the personal experience, know that that frustration, that new enlightenment about this issue, when someone close to you or yourself has to stare down that tunnel and not know if anything is going to appear. And so I think we do need an incentive. But I—obviously, it's got to be done correctly. I mean you don't want to get into the ghoulish kinds of things we've heard, those potential worst-case scenarios. I found Dr. Delmonico's testimony to probably be the most thought provoking of the day in many respects, because I sense you really come from this from your heart and have been on the end of the scalpel that matters most, and you've raised some really valid issues that cause us to think. But I sense from Dr. Sade that what you're talking about, and the AMA is talking about, isn't predetermined. You don't come in here today with a study or the plan. What you're saying is give us an opportunity to work around and see what may work within the common ethical bounds of science with a review boards approval. Is that correct?

Mr. SADE. Yeah. That's correct. I think that you can imagine the quality of research that would come out of the NIH if the NIH told the researchers, here's which projects to write and which objectives to have in their studies. I mean, you know, you wouldn't get very good science out of that. And we're trying to make this as productive and scientific a system as we possibly can, that doesn't result in a ban on all organ donation. It doesn't mean repealing the No Prohibition on Valuable Consideration. It only removes that ban for the studies that are properly designed in an ethical format and in a scientific format that will give us good information on which we can make future decisions.

Mr. WALDEN. It seems to me there'd be a real value in that if it could get done properly. I share a concern about driving the wrong incentive the wrong way. It can produce some unwelcome outcomes. But it looks to me like the more we could do to incent people to sign up and participate sooner in life, the better off we would be.

I don't know that I have any additional comments or questions. I do appreciate the testimony of all of our panelists today. You've all made us think deeper about this issue as we all struggle for the same outcome, which is to get more people to sign up to be organ donors because we know the miracle that results when they do.

Thank you Mr. Chairman.

Mr. GREENWOOD. The Chair thanks the gentleman. The Chair thanks the panel.

We have a series of votes right now, so our timing has turned out to be perfect.

Thank you. This is obviously a controversial, but important subject, and you have contributed mightily to it today. The hearing is adjourned.

[Whereupon, at 1:22 p.m., the subcommittee was adjourned.]
[Additional material submitted for the record follows:]

U.S. DEPARTMENT OF HEALTH AND HUMAN SERVICES ADVISORY COMMITTEE ON ORGAN TRANSPLANTATION

RECOMMENDATIONS TO THE SECRETARY

Following more than a year of deliberations and meetings, Secretary Tommy G. Thompson's Advisory Committee on Organ Transplantation (ACOT) met on November 18-19, 2002, in Arlington, Virginia, and unanimously agreed upon a series of consensus recommendations with respect to a number of serious organ donation and transplantation issues, affecting all recipients as well as both deceased and living donors.

The first day of that meeting was devoted by the Committee to responding to Secretary Thompson's specific request to them that they look into several concerns he had with respect to the process of live organ donation and transplantation—particularly regarding the kidney, liver and lung—so as to ensure that the donation and transplantation process would be as safe and effective as possible, for both the living organ donor and the recipient of the donor's organ.

ACOT believes that the implementation of these first seven recommendations will ensure the protection of potential living donors and simultaneously enhance the effectiveness of living donation and transplantation.

Recommendation 1: That the following ethical principles and informed consent standards be implemented for all living donors.

The Secretary's first request was that ACOT consider the desirability of national disclosure standards. ACOT responded by recommending a series of ethical principles and elements of informed consent that should be implemented for all living donors.

ACOT agrees upon a set of Ethical Principles of Consent to Being a Live Organ Donor, which includes the view that the person who gives consent to becoming a live organ donor must be:

- competent (possessing decision making capacity)
- willing to donate
- free from coercion
- medically and psychosocially suitable
- fully informed of the risks and benefits as a donor and
- fully informed of the risks, benefits, and alternative treatment available to the recipient.

Two related ethical principles that ACOT endorses are:

- Equipoise; i.e., the benefits to both the donor and the recipient must outweigh the risks associated with the donation and transplantation of the live donor organ; and
- A clear statement that the potential donor's participation must be completely voluntary, and may be withdrawn at any time.

ACOT recommends that each institution develop an informed consent document that would be understandable to all potential donors. Such a document should be accessible to people at all educational levels, and appropriate for the potential donor's level of education. Apart from the need to employ specifically defined medical terms, the document should in most circumstances be written for readers with no higher than an 8th or 9th grade level of education. If the potential donor does not speak English, there should be an independent interpreter to facilitate understanding in the patient's language. Where appropriate, translations of such a document and accompanying materials should be made available.

ACOT further recommends that the following Standards of Disclosure: Elements of Informed Consent be incorporated in the informed consent document given to the potential live organ donor, with specific descriptions that would ensure the donor's awareness of:

- the purpose of the donation
- the evaluation process—including interviews, examinations, laboratory tests, and other procedures—and the possibility that the potential donor may be found ineligible to donate
- the donation surgical procedure
- the alternative procedures or courses of treatment for potential donor and recipient
- any procedures which are or may be considered to be experimental
- the immediate recovery period and the anticipated post-operative course of care

- the foreseeable risks or discomforts to the potential donor
- the potential psychological effects resulting from the process of donation
- the reported national experience, transplant center and surgeon-specific statistics of donor outcomes, including the possibility that the donor may subsequently experience organ failure and/or disability or death
- the foreseeable risks, discomforts, and survival benefit to the potential recipient
- the reported national experience and transplant center statistics of recipient outcomes, including failure of the donated organ and the possibility of recipient death
- the fact that the potential donor's participation is voluntary, and may be withdrawn at any time
- the fact that the potential donor may derive a medical benefit by having a previously undetected health problem diagnosed as a result of the evaluation process
- the fact that the potential donor undertakes risk and derives no medical benefit from the operative procedure of donation
- the fact that unforeseen future risks or medical uncertainties may not be identifiable at the time of donation
- the fact that the potential donor may be reimbursed for the personal expenses of travel, housing, and lost wages related to donation
- the prohibition against the donor otherwise receiving any valuable consideration (including monetary or material gain) for agreeing to be a donor
- the fact that the donor's existing health and disability insurance may not cover the potential long-term costs and medical and psychological consequences of donation
- the fact that the donor's act of donation may adversely affect the donor's future eligibility for health, disability, or life insurance
- additional informational resources relating to live organ donation (possibly through the establishment of a separate resources center, as separately recommended)
- the fact that Government approved agencies and contractors will be able to obtain information regarding the donor's health for life and
- the principles of confidentiality, clarifying that:
- communication between the donor and the transplant center will remain confidential;
- a decision by the potential donor not to proceed with the donation will only be disclosed with the consent of the potential donor;
- the transplant center will share the donor's identity and other medical information with entities involved in the procurement and transplantation of organs, as well as registries that are legally charged to follow donor outcomes; and
- confidentiality of all patient information will be maintained in accord with applicable laws and regulations.

ACOT also prepared two specific informed consent documents that embody these principles and elements. The first relates to the potential donor's initial consent for evaluation as a possible donor, Living Liver Donor Initial Consent for Evaluation (appendix 1). The second deals with the potential donor's informed consent for surgery, Living Liver Donor Informed Consent for Surgery (appendix 2).

ACOT recognizes that institutions operating in different states across the nation may have different laws and needs that will affect the precise wording of the informed consent document(s) they will use. For that reason, these consent documents are submitted as examples and possible models only. Note as well that, although the specific examples are for living liver donation, ACOT is recommending such forms for all potential living organ donors.

Moreover, ACOT does not believe that these or any forms are a substitute for in-person communication between physicians and other involved professionals and the potential donor. These forms should be viewed instead as only the written evidence of discussions leading to informed consent based upon full disclosure.

Recommendation 2: That each institution that performs living donor transplantation provide an independent donor advocate to ensure that the informed consent standards and ethical principles described above are applied to the practice of all live organ donor transplantation.

The Secretary's second request was that ACOT consider the desirability of an independent donor advocate (or advocacy team) to represent and advise the donor so as to ensure that the previously described elements and ethical principles are applied to the practice of all live donor transplantation.

ACOT agrees with this principle and herein provides detailed recommendations as to how such an independent donor advocate should be established, as well as the role and qualifications of such an advocate.

ACOT recommends that each transplant center identify and provide to each potential donor an independent and trained patient advocate whose primary obligation would be to help donors understand the process, the procedure and risks and benefits of live organ donation; and to protect and promote the interests and well being of the donor.

ACOT recognizes that there is an acknowledged limitation of objectivity and independence, given the realities of the processes that take place within a transplant center among medical colleagues who regularly interact professionally; a modern, practicing physician does not work in a vacuum and cannot perform in a way that is wholly apart from other institutional staff. Moreover, the donor advocate should not be totally independent of events affecting the recipient, as there must be interaction of the advocate with the transplant surgeon of the recipient team. However, the concept of preserving a separate care physician for the donor is underscored as the reason to retain the word independent in the identity of the advocate.

Recommendation 3: That a database of health outcomes for all live donors be established and funded through and under the auspices of the U.S. Department of Health and Human Services.

The Secretary's third request was that ACOT consider the desirability of establishing a living organ donor registry. ACOT concurs with the Secretary's suggestion and recommends that a database of health outcomes of all live donors be established and further recommends that the registry or database should build upon existing smaller databases, but believes that a comprehensive national database will be necessary to answer the Secretary's desire that all potential organ donors be fully informed and aware of the likely consequences of their decisions.

The Secretary asked ACOT where such a database should be established and ACOT believes that only the Department of Health and Human Services has the authority and resources to establish such a registry. There are valid competing arguments as to what component of DHHS should have primary responsibility for funding and managing such a registry, and ACOT therefore offers no consensus suggestion on this question, but ACOT stands ready to assist the Department in further deliberations on this question.

ACOT further stands ready to assist the Secretary in suggesting information or data elements (and the time periods for the collection of such data) that should be included in such a registry, but it was felt that further discussions within the Department, and with the OPTN, as well as with the SRTR, would be necessary, given ACOT's understanding that the substantial cost implications in establishing and maintaining such a registry must be fully explored.

In order to guide Departmental deliberations on those questions, ACOT responds to the Secretary's request for its opinion on how the information collected should be used. ACOT believes that the primary purpose of such a registry should be to enable the medical community to define accurately the donor risks and benefits of live organ transplantation so as to give potential donors an accurate risk assessment.

Recommendation 4: That serious consideration be given to the establishment of a separate resource center for living donors and their families.

ACOT recommends advancing the information and resources available to living donors and their families through the implementation of detailed consent forms, the creation of independent donor advocates and the establishment of a living donor registry. To similar effect, ACOT recommends the establishment of a separate office, a resource center, for potential living donors, those who choose to donate, as well as their families. The primary function of such a resource center would be to ensure that each potential donor receives a complete and current set of information about living organ donation.

An existing model for such a resource center is in place at the OPTN, which has both a person to contact for information, and a web site with information specific to the needs of transplant candidates and recipients. The resource center could either be located under the aegis of the OPTN or the living donor registry. Such a distinct resource center would have the benefit of being clearly distinguished as separate and apart from the transplant team and hospital. Until such time as such an independent resource center is established, ACOT recommends that transplant centers should give consideration to providing such a resource center on their own, again with the purpose of ensuring that each potential donor receives a complete and current set of information about living organ donation.

Recommendation 5: That the present preference in OPTN allocation policy—given to prior living organ donors who subsequently need a kidney—be extended so that any living organ donor would be given preference as a candidate for any organ transplant, should one become needed.

This recommendation states that there should be a preference accorded to the living organ donor. The point value or other means of assigning such a preference is left to the OPTN.

Recommendation 6: That the requirements for HLA typing of liver transplant recipients and/or living liver donors should be deleted.

This testing may, however, be appropriate for some donors and recipients and in such cases should be compensated by Medicaid, Medicare or private insurers as appropriate, when specifically ordered, as for all other appropriate laboratory tests.

Recommendation 7: that a process be established that would verify the qualifications of a center to perform living donor liver or lung transplantation.

ACOT believes that a process needs to be established that would verify the qualifications of a center to perform living donor liver or lung transplantation. ACOT believes that the process for performing living kidney transplantation is sufficiently mature and established that no further verification processes are required. ACOT believes that, owing to the relative newness of the procedures, as well as the inherent intricacies of the operations, that centers performing and seeking to perform living donor liver and living donor lung transplantation each require further review and verification within the medical community.

The purpose of such a verification process would be to give patients an increased level of confidence in the institutions performing such operations, and to provide a guide for centers seeking to enter this field.

Although the Secretary's recent letters to the Committee have focused on living donation, his overall charge to the Committee has been much broader, and ACOT has responded to that charge by promulgating an additional series of recommendations not specific to living donation.

The second day of the ACOT meeting was devoted by the Committee to issues affecting equitable access to transplantation, and those relating to deceased or cadaveric donors.

ACOT believes that the implementation of the following two recommendations, which relate to access to transplantation, will especially benefit minority populations.

Recommendation 8: That specific methods be employed to increase the education and awareness of patients at dialysis centers as to transplant options available to them.

Available information indicates that too many patients at dialysis centers are unaware of the transplant options available to them. Too many of these patients are members of minority groups. Given the cost of sustained dialysis treatment, both to patients and to the Centers for Medicare and Medicaid Services, as compared to the cost of transplantation, this would also be cost-effective as well as life-saving.

In order to assure the accuracy of this assessment, ACOT recommends that procedural methodologies be developed to evaluate dialysis patient access and referral for organ transplant, as well as an accurate cost/benefit analysis, using existing data and/or new sources of data.

ACOT further recommends that, as soon as possible, a health education program be implemented, and/or that an educational coordinator be placed on site at individual dialysis centers so as to provide patients with adequate education about transplant options available to them. This would be a reinforcement of the implementation of existing regulations stipulating that dialysis patients be educated and evaluated by personnel from the transplant center concerning this therapeutic option.

Recommendation 9: That research be conducted into the causes of existing disparities in organ transplant rates and outcomes, with the goal of eliminating those disparities.

The fact of such disparities, particularly with regard to kidney transplantation rates, appears to be undisputed, and data developed by the SRTR for ACOT highlights this issue. HRSA, NIH and other DHHS agencies are presently committed to research aimed at ending such disparities with respect to health care delivery in other areas, and research should be undertaken to establish whether any separate reasons may exist for such disparities within the transplantation area, and, if so, how they may be eliminated.

ACOT believes that the implementation of the following nine recommendations, which primarily relate to increasing the supply of deceased donor organs, will ultimately, and in some cases very quickly, mean many more additional organs becoming available to potential recipients.

Recommendation 10: That legislative strategies be adopted that will encourage medical examiners and coroners not to withhold life-saving organs and tissues from qualified organ procurement organizations.

Studies indicate that coroners and medical examiners across the United States are not uniform in their approach to making organs available to organ procurement organizations, and that many unnecessarily withhold from retrieval organs that could be used for transplantation. Indeed, it is estimated that if all states followed the example of Texas, which has enacted a law containing a provision similar to the one below, then 700-1,000 additional organs would be made additionally available each year.

The Secretary is specifically encouraged to use his good standing with the National Governor's Association, the National Association of State Legislatures, the Uniform Commissioners of State Laws, and/or with individual states to seek the following change:

To amend the Uniform Anatomical Gift Act (UAGA) to add a new subsection at the end of section 4, as follows:

(d) If the medical examiner is considering withholding one or more organs or tissues of a potential donor for any reason, the medical examiner shall be present during the removal of the organs or tissue. In such case, the medical examiner may request a biopsy of those organs or tissue, or deny their removal. If the medical examiner denies removal of any organ or tissue, the medical examiner shall explain in writing the reasons for the denial and shall provide the explanation to the qualified organ procurement organization.

In the alternative, the Secretary is asked to encourage individual states to adopt state laws to the same or similar effect.

Recommendation 11: That the secretary of HHS, in concert with the Secretary of Education, should recommend to states that organ and tissue donation be included in core curriculum standards for public education as well as in the curricula of professional schools, including schools of education, schools of medicine, schools of nursing, schools of law, schools of public health, schools of social work, and pharmacy schools.

The Secretary of HHS, in collaboration with the Secretary of Education, should identify relevant core curriculum standards, and survey those courses and curricula that presently include education as to organ and tissue donation, with a view to promoting a model standard that can be broadly employed in public education. This would, at a minimum, include all high schools.

In addition, hospitals should establish ongoing basic introductory (new hire) programs, focused on organ and tissue donation that would be similar to CPR certification and recertification, and might in fact be accommodated within the same new hire program.

Efforts should also be made to ensure that organ and tissue donation be a part of the professional educational curricula at all professional schools related to health. Law schools are included because of the relevance of such issues to courses in elder law, estate planning, and health law.

Recommendation 12: That in order to ensure best practices, organ procurement organizations and the OPTN be encouraged to develop, evaluate, and support the implementation of improved management protocols of potential donors.

This recommendation builds upon those made at previous conferences held by various transplantation related organizations, as well as work performed under contract to the Department. A novel and improved standard of titrated care for heart and lung donors has been established and ACOT believes that it should be more generally implemented. It is known as the Critical Pathway for the Organ Donor (appendix 3, .pdf—get the free Reader). Similar improved standards of management and care should be developed to optimize the potential recovery of other organs.

Recommendation 13: That in order to ensure best practices at hospitals and organ procurement organizations, the following measure should be added to the CMS conditions of participation: each hospital with more than 100 beds should identify an advocate for organ and tissue donation from within the hospital clinical staff.

Such a designated advocate for organ and tissue donation would be responsible for assuring that the facility is in compliance with the Conditions of Participation as well as any other policies that pertain to organ and tissue donation. In addition, this designated advocate's responsibilities would include assuring that efforts are made to promote donation in the local community. (Given varying hospital management structures, such an advocate may not always be a member of the clinical staff; what is essential, however, is that the advocate have the institutional authority to effect change.)

Recommendation 14: That in order to ensure best practices at hospitals and organ procurement organizations, the following measure should be added to the CMS conditions of participation: Each hospital should estab-

lish, in conjunction with its OPO, policies and procedures to manage and maximize organ retrieval from donors without a heartbeat.

Such donation is often referred to as donation after cardiac death, and such donors are variously referred to as donors without a heartbeat or non-heart-beating donors, These policies and procedures will need to be developed in collaboration with the OPTN, the transplant centers and AOPO.

Recommendation 15: That the following measure be added to the CMS conditions of participation: Hospitals shall notify organ procurement organizations prior to the withdrawal of life support to a patient, so as to determine that patient's potential for organ donation. If it is determined that the patient is a potential donor, the OPO shall reimburse the hospital for appropriate costs related to maintaining that patient as a potential donor.

Recommendation 16: That the regulatory framework provided by CMS for transplant center and Organ Procurement Organization certification should be based on principles of continuous quality improvement. Subsequent failure to meet performance standards established under such principles should trigger quality improvement processes under the supervision of HRSA.

The relevant committee of the OPTN is encouraged to develop baseline measures/ principles to guide the process of continuous quality improvement, a part of which process is the development of baseline measures. The quality improvement process envisioned by ACOT might resemble one that is presently utilized in some hospitals/ facilities, and known as FOCUS-PDCA (appendix 4).

Recommendation 17: That all hospitals, particularly those with more than one hundred beds, be strongly encouraged by CMS and AHRQ to implement policies such that the failure to identify a potential organ donor and/or refer such a potential donor to the organ procurement organization in a timely manner be considered a serious medical error. Such events should be investigated and reviewed by hospitals in a manner similar to that for other major adverse healthcare events.

This measure could be added to the sort of physician profile which most facilities currently employ. (See example physician profile (appendix 5, .pdf—get the free Reader). ACOT expects that this Recommendation will have its greatest impact at those hospitals with trauma centers, as well as those with residency programs and/ or academic affiliations.

Recommendation 18: That the Joint Commission on Accreditation of Healthcare Organizations (JCAHO) strengthen its accreditation provisions regarding organ donation, including consideration of treating as a sentinel event the failure of hospitals to identify a potential donor and/or refer a donor to the relevant Organ Procurement Organization in a timely manner. Similar review should be considered by the National Committee on Quality Assurance (NCQA).

JCAHO presently defines and identifies a sentinel event as: *An unexpected occurrence involving death or serious physical or psychological injury, or the risk thereof. Serious injury specifically includes loss of limb or function. The phrase, "or the risk thereof" includes any process variation for which a recurrence would carry a significant chance of a serious adverse outcome. Such events are called "sentinel" because they signal the need for immediate investigation and response.*

Failing to identify or refer a potential donor in a timely manner carries the serious risk of that donor's organs not being made available to a potential recipient. Given the shortage of organs and the fact of so many potential recipients dying while awaiting the possibility of transplantation, such a failure would appear to fall within the JCAHO definition of a sentinel event

Monitoring hospitals for compliance with organ donation standards should become an integral part of the JCAHO hospital survey process. In addition to examination of the standard, the hospital JCAHO survey should include the OPO referral records which are submitted back to the hospital, as well as the supporting documentation of corrective measures or follow-up. There should be a compliance benchmark set (e.g., 90-100%), with anything below that benchmark requiring a gap analysis.

———

May 19, 2003

Dear Honorable Members of Congress,

The problem is simple and stark. While transplant surgery has become progressively more routine, every year tens of thousands of organs (50 to 75 percent of those potentially available) that could restore the health and prolong the lives of Americans are instead being taken to the grave, unutilized. At the same time, about 6,000 Americans die each year while waiting for organs that never arrive, in most cases after years of incredible suffering endured by themselves, their families, and their friends.

Were the failure to retrieve these vital and irreplaceable organs the result of deeply felt religious or cultural beliefs, we would not be writing to you. It is not. The only thing that stands in the way of retrieving these organs and saving many thousands of lives each year is a failure of the collective imagination—a failure to devise a policy that, while respecting traditional social norms, provides an increased incentive for cadaveric organ donation.

We believe we have a compromise plan that both comports with human dignity, and constitutes the tiniest imaginable step toward utilizing the power of financial incentives to bring the supply of cadaveric organs up to meet the demand. All available evidence suggests that such incentives will be as effective in this sphere of human need as they are in supplying all other products and services that we value. Please note that we are not proposing any change in the current system of organ allocation.

We write to you as a diverse group of academics from the legal, economic, philosophic and scientific communities who have written and spoken on this question over the years. Also joining us are transplant surgeons and leaders of Organ Procurement Organizations (OPOs) with many years of experience on the front lines of organ procurement. Our ranks also include actively interested citizens and religious and civic leaders. We are all persuaded that a properly designed system of financial incentives for cadaveric organs is likely to have a powerful salutary effect on alleviating human suffering, and we think the time has come to begin pilot studies of such a system.

We offer a consensus proposal that, we believe, will result in an almost immediate and substantial increase in the rate of cadaveric organ donation. We believe it constitutes the most viable compromise between using the power of market forces to satisfy human need while at the same time recognizing the widespread reluctance to having human body parts being treated, undignifiedly, as commodities.

The proposal involves the partial lifting of Public Law 98-507, Title III, Section 301, the section of the National Organ Transplant Act of 1984 forbidding financial incentives, insofar as it applies to cadaveric donation. Specifically, we propose that Congress instruct the Secretary of the Department of Health and Human Services to initiate demonstration projects of a policy that rewards the estates of brain-dead donors with a set donation of, for example, $5,000, for the decision of their family to give the gift of life. This policy would be instituted by the currently existing OPOs. The gift could be used to help pay for funeral or hospital costs, as a donation to the deceased's favorite charity, or could simply remain with the estate. We even propose specific language the OPO personnel could use, after their normal humanitarian appeal, in order properly to convey to families the nature of the decision they are being asked to make and of the gift they are being offered:

> *Dear Mr. Smith/Mrs. Jones, as you may know, it is our standard policy to offer a gift of $5,000 to the estate of the deceased, as a way of saying "Thank you for giving the gift of life." The money can be used to help offset funeral or hospital expenses, to donate to your loved one's favorite charity, or simply to remain with the estate, to be used in any manner the heirs see fit. No price can be placed upon the many lives that can be saved by your gift. Our donation in return is merely society's way of honoring the sacrifice you are being asked to make, and is a token of our deep and sincere appreciation for your generosity at this most difficult time.*

A crucial aspect of the proposal is that the gift be a set amount that is given to the estates of all brain-dead patients who are judged to be good donor candidates, and whose families do indeed donate. There should be no possibility of unseemly haggling. Neither should there be any reduction of the amount of the gift if a presumptively good donor turns out to have few or no usable vital organs. We think this approach would avoid, as much as possible, any slippage from a system that maintains human organs in a category wholly separate from all other, more mundane, commodities.

A second crucial aspect of the proposal is that the amount of the gift be large enough so that the family members do not feel as though the memory of their loved one is being insulted or their loss trivialized, or that they are being asked to allow themselves to be taken advantage of, especially in the hospital environment, where surgeons and top hospital administrators are known to make high six-figure salaries. We feel that $5,000 is a round and respectful sum that tangibly conveys a sense of the grave importance we as a society place upon the decision the family is being asked to make. In any case, we do not think the fixed gift amount should be less than $3,000.

This proposal is, we believe, the smallest and most effective step that can be taken away from our current system, which relies purely on altruism, to a policy that allows something of a quid pro quo—a reward for community service, much like the death benefits that currently are provided to the families of service personnel who die in the line of duty.

We note that if our proposal is successful in doubling or tripling the rate of cadaveric organ donation, as is well within the realm of possibility, our nation's deadly organ shortage would become a life-saving surplus, the growing problem of black market payments for living organ donation would largely disappear, and surgeons would have much less occasion for compromising their Hippocratic oath by endangering the lives of healthy donors.

Additionally, we note that if the project is successful, it will eventually more than pay for itself in terms of reduced dialysis expenditures by the federal End-Stage Renal Disease Program.

As you may also know, the American Medical Association, at their 2002 annual meeting, advocated experimenting with allowing compensation for cadaveric organ donation. The American Society of Transplant Surgeons and the United Network for Organ Sharing—the organization that operates the organ allocation system in the United States—have made similar proposals.— But, none of these proposals can proceed without someone in Congress taking charge to amend current law.

If, as we fervently hope, you do wish to redress this tragic situation, we are available to meet and discuss it with you or your staff at your convenience. Every moment we delay, more untold suffering occurs and more Americans die needlessly. The time to act is now.

Sincerely, Signed (in alphabetical order)

FATHER PHILLIP L. ADAMS, *Minister and Director, Lighthouse Christian Ministries; Richard Amerling, M.D., Nephrologist, Beth Israel Medical Center of New York, Albert Einstein College of Medicine;* BRIAN A. BROZNICK, *President and CEO, Center for Organ Recovery & Education (CORE);* CHARLES T. CARLSTROM, PH.D., *Economic Advisor, Federal Reserve Bank of Cleveland;* FATHER JOHN CHAKOS, *Priest, Holy Cross Greek Orthodox Church;* LLOYD COHEN, J.D., PH.D., *Professor, George Mason University School of Law;* REVEREND GARY W. DENNING, *Minister, First Baptist Church of Pittsburgh;* RICHARD A. EPSTEIN, *James Parker Hall Distinguished Service Professor of Law, University of Chicago, Peter and Kirsten Bedford Senior Fellow, Hoover Institution;* JOHN J. FUNG, M.D., PH.D. *Thomas E. Starzl Professor of Transplantation Surgery and Chief, Division of Transplant Surgery, University of Pittsburgh School of Medicine, Director, Thomas E. Starzl Transplantation Institute, Board Member, United Network for Organ Sharing (UNOS);* RABBI MEL GOTTLIEB, PH.D., *Dean, Academy for Jewish Religion;* DAVID L. KASERMAN, PH.D., *Torchmark Professor of Economics, Department of Economics, Auburn University;* BABURAO KONERU, M.D., *Associate Professor and Chief, Division of Transplant Surgery, New Jersey Medical School-Newark, University of Medicine and Dentistry of New Jersey, Former Board Member, New Jersey Organ & Tissue Sharing Network;* HAROLD KYRIAZI, PH.D., *Research Associate, Department of Neurobiology, University of Pittsburgh School of Medicine;* MERRILL MATTHEWS JR., PH.D., *Director, Council for Affordable Health Insurance;* GREGORY PENCE, PH.D., *Medical Ethicist, School of Medicine and Department of Philosophy, University of Alabama at Birmingham;* THOMAS G. PETERS, M.D., *Director, Jacksonville Transplant Center, Shands Jacksonville Medical Center, Former Board Member, UNOS;* WILLIAM RUSSELL ROBINSON, *7-term member, Pennsylvania State House of Representatives 1989-2003, Sponsor, Pennsylvania Organ Donor Trust Fund legislation, Sponsor, state legislation authorizing $300 funeral benefit for organ donor families, Member, Pittsburgh City Council, 1978-1985;* ROBERT M. SADE, M.D., *Professor, Dept. of Surgery, Medical University of South Carolina, Medical Director, LifePoint, Inc., Director, Institute of Human Values in Health Care, Member, UNOS Ethics Committee, Member, AMA Council on Ethical and Judicial Affairs;* LAWRENCE L. SCHKADE, PH.D., CCP, *Garrett Professor of Information Systems, University of Texas-Arlington, Heart Transplant Recipient, 1992, Member, UNOS Board of Directors, Member, Board of Directors, LifeGift Organ Donation Center;* ALEXANDER TABARROK, PH.D., *Professor, Department of Economics, George Mason University, Director of Research, The Independent Institute;* MARK THORNTON, PH.D., *Economist, Ludwig von Mises Institute;* and DAVID J. UNDIS, *Executive Director, LifeSharers.*

June 6, 2003

The Honorable JIM GREENWOOD
Chairman
Subcommittee on Oversight and Investigations
Energy and Commerce Committee
U.S. House of Representatives
Washington, DC 20515

The Honorable PETER DEUTSCH
Ranking Member
Subcommittee on Oversight and Investigations
Energy and Commerce Committee
U.S. House of Representatives
Washington, DC 20515

Dear CHAIRMAN GREENWOOD and RANKING MEMBER DEUTSCH: On June 2, 2003, I testified on behalf of the American Society of Transplant Surgeons (ASTS) during the hearing entitled "Assessing Initiatives to Increase Organ Donations."

In written testimony submitted to the Subcommittee during the hearing, the American Medical Association's Robert M. Sade, MD, made a statement that included the following:

> "Models have been proposed by several organizations, including ASTS and UNOS, whose Board of Directors agreed, days after the AMA adopted its policy, to support legislation that would enable studying the impact of incentives to encourage organ donation and to honor organ donors. Among the suggested models are: future contracts, as was proposed in a bill before Congress several years ago, that would have *allowed for the implementation of a tax credit of up to $10,000 on the estate of the deceased donor*; reimbursement for funeral expenses, as was passed into law in Pennsylvania, but was never implemented because of the federal prohibition..."

ASTS would like to correct this statement for the record. At no time did the ASTS endorse a tax credit of $10,000 on the estate of the deceased donor. The AMA testimony is correct, however, that ASTS endorsed a study on the concept of reimbursement for funeral expenses.

Thank you for allowing us the opportunity to testify at the hearing on these and other important issues relating to organ donation. We look forward to working with you and your Subcommittee in the future on this issue. If you have any questions, please contact Peter W. Thomas, ASTS's Legislative Counsel, at (202) 466-6550.

Sincerely,

ABRAHAM SHAKED, M.D., PH.D.
President

cc: Robert M. Sade, MD, American Medical Association

ETHICAL OPINION ON "THE RICHARD M. DE VOS POSITION PAPER ON FINANCIAL INCENTIVES FOR ORGAN DONATION"

DR. SAMUEL GREGG, ACTON INSTITUTE

April 17, 2003*

SITUATION

1. The progress and spread of transplant medicine and surgery nowadays makes possible treatment and cure for many illnesses which, up to a short time ago, could only lead to death or, at best, a painful and limited existence. This "service to life," [1] which the donation and transplant of organs represents, shows its moral value and legitimizes its medical practice. There are, however, some conditions which must be observed, particularly those regarding donors and the organs donated and implanted. Every organ or human tissue transplant requires an explant which in some way impairs the corporeal integrity of the donor.

2. The present shortage of available organs for transplant has resulted in a number of propositions for improving the situation so as to preserve the life of those in

---

*Copyright 2002© by Samuel Gregg. For permission to cite, reproduce or circulate this paper, please contact the author at sgregg@acton.org, or Acton Institute, 161 Ottawa Ave NW, Suite 301, Grand Rapids, MI 49503, USA. Ph. 1-616-454-3080

[1] John Paul II, "To the participants at the First International Congress on the Transplant of Organs," June 20, 1991, in *Insegnamenti*, XIV/1 (1991), p. 1710.

danger of imminent death, and/or to improve the health of those who are suffering from various ailments. These propositions range from state-funding of more Organ Donation coordinators, to the establishment of a free market in organs.

3. Not all options, however, are morally acceptable. Moreover, every option must be subject to clear, coherent and rationally defensible ethical analysis. The approach used in this opinion is that of the authoritative moral teaching of the Magisterium of the Roman Catholic Church and the natural law tradition (specifically that articulated by the Magisterium). It does so on the basis that (a) all other approaches that purport to be based on reason alone are essentially deficient and ultimately incoherent; and (b) that the moral truth of natural law is, by definition, accessible to all. The Church thus rejects those approaches to morality, such as all forms of utilitarianism, that require people to engage in the epistemologically and intellectually impossible task of measuring and weighing all the certain and possible good and evil effects of an action.[2] To cite John Paul II, "How could an absolute obligation resulting from such debatable calculations be justified?"[3] Instead, the Catholic analysis of a policy's moral dimension focuses upon asking whether an option is choiceworthy, or if it is excluded from upright choice by its opposition in some way to the human goods (bona humana) to which St. Thomas Aquinas says all people, religious or otherwise, are directed by the first principles of practical reasonableness,[4] the basic reasons for action which the encyclical letter Veritatis Splendor calls "fundamental human goods."[5]

4. This opinion considers only one proposition: that is, "The Richard M. De Vos Position Paper on Financial Incentives for Organ Donation" (hereafter the Position Paper). This proposition involves the establishment of a tax incentive or an insurance benefit to be received by the designated beneficiary of a donor upon the successful transplant of the donor's organs following the donor's natural death. This policy encourages people to designate, unambiguously, if they wish to have their organs recovered after death with the object of an act being the saving of human life.

5. Should there be any change in the composition of the Position Paper, this opinion should be considered null and void until the author has had the opportunity to consider the ethical implications of the changes.

6. Should the Magisterium of the Roman Catholic Church pronounce authoritatively and specifically on the proposition articulated in the Position Paper or a similar proposition, then the author's position should be henceforth assumed to adhere to that of the Church.

THE CATHOLIC POSITION ON ORGAN TRANSPLANTATION AND COMPENSATION FOR DONATION OF HUMAN ORGANS

There are positive and negative dimensions to the teaching of the Catholic Church on organ transplantation and the question of compensation.

Positive Dimensions

1. Transplantation between species, specifically from animal to human, in general, is not morally forbidden. "It cannot be said that every transplant of tissues (biologically possible) between two individuals of different species is morally reprehensible, but it is even less true that every heterogeneous transplant biologically possible is not forbidden and cannot raise objections. A distinction must be made between cases, depending on which tissue or organ is intended for transplant. The transplant of animal sexual glands to humans must be rejected as immoral; but the transplant of the cornea of a non-human organism to a human organism would not create any problem if it were biologically possible and advisable."[6]

---

[2] See John Finnis, *Fundamentals of Ethics* (Washington, D.C.: Georgetown University Press, 1983): pp.86-94.

[3] See John Paul II, Encyclical Letter *Veritatis Splendor,* 1993, para. 77.

[4] In Aquinas's words, "The good of the human being is being in accord with reason, and human evil is being outside the order of reasonableness." ST, I-II, q.71, a.2. Or, as Aquinas states elsewhere, "good is the first thing that falls under the apprehension of the practical reason, which is directed to action: since every agent acts for an end under the aspect of good. Consequently the first principle in the practical reason is one founded on the notion of good." ST, I-II, q.94, a.2. Thus for Aquinas, the way to discover what is morally right (virtue) and wrong (vice) is to ask, not what is in accordance with human nature, but what is reasonable. See John Finnis, *Natural Law and Natural Rights* (Oxford: Clarendon Press, 1980), p.36; and Samuel Gregg, *Morality, Law, and Public Policy* (Sydney: St. Thomas More Press, 2001), p.23.

[5] *Veritatis Splendor,* para.48.

[6] Pius XII, "To the delegates of the Italian Association of Cornea Donors and the Italian Union for the Blind", May 14, 1956, *AAS* 48 (1956): pp. 462-464.

2. Transplantation from a corpse requires that the corpse be treated with the respect due to the abode of a spiritual and immortal soul, an essential constituent of a human person whose dignity it shared.[7]

3. Transplantation from a corpse to a living being is permissible. Physicians should not, however, be permitted to undertake excisions or other operations on a corpse without the permission of those charged with its care and perhaps even in the face of objections previously expressed by the person in question.[8] "Organ transplants are not morally acceptable if the donor or those who legitimately speak for him have not given their informed consent. Organ transplants conform with the moral law and can be meritorious if the physical and psychological dangers and risks incurred by the donor are proportionate to the good sought for the recipient. It is morally inadmissible directly to bring about the disabling mutilation or death of a human being, even in order to delay the death of other persons."[9]

4. People may choose in their wills to dispose of their bodies after natural death for legitimate medical purposes.[10]

5. Organ transplantation from a live donor is also permissible. People are not, however, free to destroy or mutilate their members or in any other way render themselves unfit for their natural functions, except when no other provision can be made for the good of the whole body. This does not rule out live organ donation for transplantation, provided that the donor's own health, identity, or adequate biological functioning is not endangered. "One can donate only what he can deprive himself of without serious danger to his life or personal identity, and for a just and proportionate reason."[11] Vital organs may only be donated after death.[12]

6. Organ donation is neither a duty nor "an obligatory act of charity."[13] But "a transplant, and even a simple blood transfusion, is not like other operations. It must not be separated from the donor's act of self-giving, from the love that gives life. The physician should always be conscious of the particular nobility of this work; he becomes the mediator of something especially significant, the *gift of self* which one person has made—even after death—so that another might live."[14]

7. Specifically regarding the issue of incentives for organ donation, compensation (financial or otherwise) is not in principle ruled out. "In advertising (for cornea donors) an intelligent reserve should be maintained to avoid serious interior and exterior conflicts. Also, is it necessary, as often happens, to refuse any compensation as a matter of principle? The question has arisen. Without doubt there can be grave abuses if recompense is demanded; but it would be an exaggeration to say that any acceptance or requirement of recompense is immoral. The case is analogous to that of blood transfusion; it is to the donor's credit if he refuses recompense, but it is not necessarily a fault to accept it."[15] Hence, while organ donation is commendable, acceptance of compensation may be permissible.

Negative Dimensions

1. The following conditions would render compensation for donating human organs morally impermissible: (a) if the compensation were carried out in a manner that obfuscates, denies, or undermines the belief in the divine origin of human life or the dignity thereby due the corpse; (b) if the intention and object of seeking compensation for either oneself or others was an illegal, immoral, or irreligious end, or directly violated one or more of the fundamental human goods; or (c) the act of compensation amounted to merely instrumentalising the donor or the donor's mere self-instrumentalization.

2. The transplantation of the sexual glands from animals to humans is to be rejected as immoral [16] because such a transplant would directly deny the sacred element in humanity and the goods of human love.

3. Society, specifically in the form of its political organization, the State, may not commandeer the organs of a deceased human being without the prior permission of

---

[7] See Pius XII, *Papal Teachings: The Human Body* (Boston, MA: Daughters of St. Paul, 1960), p.380.

[8] See Pius XII, *Papal Teachings: The Human Body* (Boston: Daughters of St. Paul, 160), p.379, p.382.

[9] *Catechism of the Catholic Church,* para. 2296.

[10] See Pius XII, *Papal Teachings: The Human Body,* p.381

[11] John Paul II, "To the participants at the First International Congress on the Transplant of Organs," p. 1711.

[12] See John Paul II, "Many Ethical, Legal, and Social Questions must be examined in greater depth," *Dolentium Hominum,* June 1991: pp.12-13.

[13] Pius XII, *Papal Teachings: The Human Body,* p.381.

[14] John Paul II, "To the participants at the First International Congress on the Transplant of Organs," p. 1711.

[15] Pius XII, *Papal Teachings: The Human Body,* p.381.

[16] See Pius XII, *Papal Teachings: The Human Body,* p.374.

that person or the consent of his family.[17] The relation of individual human persons to the body politic is moral, not organic. This rules out any form of coercive donation, including organ procurement strategies such as presumed consent in which, absent a specific refusal, one is presumed to have consented to donation.

4. It is forbidden for any form of organ donation, be it by a living donor or from a corpse, to involve any mere instrumentalization of the person from whom the organ is taken. This prohibition includes any mere self-instrumentalization by a living donor. John Paul II states, "The body cannot be treated as a merely physical or biological entity, nor can its organs ever be used as items of sale or exchange. Such a reductive materialist conception would lead to a merely instrumental use of the body and therefore of the person. In such a perspective, organ transplantation and the grating of tissue would no longer correspond to an act of donation but would amount to the dispossession or plundering of the body."[18] Acceptance of compensation for oneself or others, as described above, however, need not proceed from a choice merely to instrumentalise oneself.

5. It is forbidden to engage in the commercial trafficking of bodies. "Also, in the case of dead fetuses, as for the corpses of adult persons, all commercial trafficking must be considered illicit and should be prohibited."[19]

6. "Ethically, not all organs can be donated. The brain and the gonads may not be transplanted because they ensure the personal and procreative identity respectively. These are organs which embody the characteristic uniqueness of the person, which medicine is bound to protect."[20]

ANALYSIS

1. The policy outlined in the Position Paper does not appear to violate any of the negative precepts of the moral teaching of the Roman Catholic Church. This is critical as the Church has always taught that it is never permissible to do evil that good may come of it.[21] St. Augustine among others notes the idea that one may do evil that good may come was something "which...the Apostle Paul detested."[22] While the positive moral precepts of the Church's teaching allow room for prudence, the negative moral precepts do not allow for legitimate exception.[23]

2. The Position Paper does not violate any of the points listed under the Positive Dimension. It would appear to fall under the legitimate compensation position stated in point 7 of the Positive Dimension. While it is to the donor's credit if he permits particular organs to be used after his death (in accordance with the guidelines outlined above) without compensation, it is not necessarily a fault to direct compensation for the use of such organs to designated beneficiaries.

3. The Position Paper does not violate any of the points listed under the Negative Dimension. The family of the deceased may, for example, still object to the removal of organs, though this would nullify any insurance benefit or monetary compensation. Nor does the Position Paper amount to allowing the use of organs as items of sale and exchange.

4. It is very important that the Position Paper uses the word *compensation* when defining the nature of any form of monetary payment. It should also specify that any organs gathered under this proposition would not consequently be sold or used as items of exchange by either the family or the institution paying the compensation. This will prevent any violations of points 4 and 5 of the Negative Dimension of the Church's teaching about organ donation and compensation.

---

[17] See Pius XII, *Papal Teachings: The Human Body*, p.376.

[18] John Paul II, "Blood and Organ Donors, August 2, 1984," *The Pope Speaks* Vol.30, no.1, 1985: pp.1-2.

[19] Congregation for the Doctrine of the Faith, Instruction on Respect for Human Life in its Origin and on the Dignity of Procreation—Replies to certain questions of the day, *Donum vitae*, 1987, I, 4.

[20] Pontifical Council for Pastoral Assistance, "Guidelines for Health Care Workers," 1 April 1996, para.88.

[21] See Rm 3:8; 1 Co 6:9-10.

[22] St. Augustine, *Contra mendacium*, i. 1.

[23] See *Veritatis Splendor*, para.52: "The negative precepts of the natural law are universally valid. They oblige each and every individual, always and in each circumstance...the negative commandments oblige always and under all circumstances...The Church has always taught that one may never choose kinds of behavior prohibited by the moral commandments expressed in negative form in the Old and New Testaments."

APEX
TP_CF
9780160708275

76523826 -- 28